THE IRISH BETTER BIRTH BOOK

THE IRISH BETTER BIRTH BOOK

Taking the Mystery (and Fear) Out of Childbirth

Tracy Donegan

The Liffey Press

Published by
The Liffey Press
Ashbrook House, 10 Main Street,
Raheny, Dublin 5, Ireland
www.theliffeypress.com

A catalogue record of this book is
available from the British Library.

ISBN 978-1-908308-08-5

Printed in the Republic of Ireland by Gemini International.

Contents

About the Author   *x*

Acknowledgements   *xi*

Introduction   **1**

Why This Book?   1

Fear-Free Birth   2

How to Use This Book   4

    Do-it-Yourself Childbirth   *6*

You're Pregnant! What Now?   **11**

The First Antenatal Visit   12

Antenatal Classes   13

    Dumb Excuses Not to Take Antenatal Classes   *15*

Ultrasound Scans   17

Making the Best Choices for You and Your Baby   **20**

What About my Baby?   20

    Take a Baby Bonding Break Today!   *21*

    Therese's Birth Story   *22*

    Ann's Birth Story   *24*

Evidence-Based Care   30

    Fish Can't See Water   *31*

    Informed Decision Making, Informed Consent and

    Informed Refusal   *33*

How to Choose your Caregiver   37

Choosing a Hospital   42

    Ten Questions to Ask Your Hospital   *42*

    Grainne's First Birth Experience   *46*

    Louise's Birth Story   *48*

Choosing Your Birth Partner   52

The Fear Factor   53

Your Birth Preferences   54

    Sample Birth Preferences   *58*

Helping Yourself to Complementary Therapies   59
Antenatal Massage   59
Acupuncture/Acupressure   60
Aromatherapy in Pregnancy   60
Herbal Use for Pregnancy and Birth   62
Bach Flower Remedies   63
Homeopathy   64
GentleBirth   65
Active Birth or Yoga Classes   65
Gentle Exercises During Pregnancy   66

Labour: Is This It?   69
Labour: Recognising the Signs   69
What to Bring to the Hospital   74
Induction   76

Pain Management in Labour   80
Methods of Managing Pain   81
    The Secret to an Easier Birth: How your
    Hormones Affect Birth   84
Old School Childbirth   86
Ways to Be Active During Labour   88
Using Pain Management Techniques   92
GentleBirth   92
    HypnoBirthing: Sara's Birth Story   96
Labour is Good for Babies!   98
Positions for Birth   99

Routine Medical Interventions   102
Failure to Progress or Failure to Wait?   102
Amniotomy (Rupturing your Membranes)   103
Eating in Labour – Why It's Good for You and Your Baby   105
Epidural   108
Monitoring Your Baby   111
Episiotomy   112
    Episiotomy: Myths and Realities   114
Delayed Cord Clamping   115
Other Interventions   117
Learning How to Push   120
Cascade of Intervention   122

Multiple Births   **123**
What if it's Twins?   123
Possible Complications   123

When Things Aren't Going to Plan   **126**
Big Baby Syndrome   126
CPD? Don't Panic!   *126*
What if My Baby is Breech?   128
Vincent's Breech Birth – First Time Mum   *128*
Jennifer's Birth Story – Second Baby   *134*
Breech Birth: What Are Your Options?   *143*
What if My Baby is in the Posterior Position?   145
Tips for Turning a Posterior Baby Before Labour   *146*

Caesarean Section   **148**
Please Read Me!   148
When is it Necessary?   148
What Normally Happens During a Caesarean?   150
Risks of Caesarean Section   *152*
Immediate Care After a Caesarean   153
Tips for Recovery After a Caesarean   *153*
Choosing a Caesarean   155
A Positive Caesarean   *156*
Caesarean Birth Plan   *159*
Baby Leon's Arrival   *159*
VBAC: Vaginal Birth After Caesarean   163
Questions about VBAC   *164*
Carolan's Birth Story   *166*

The Times They Are a-Changin':
New Developments in Maternity Care   **172**
Domino Scheme   172
Early Transfer Home Scheme   173
Midwife-Led Services   173
Doulas Do What?   175

Giving Birth at Home   **176**
The Modern McBirth   *177*
Home Birth Care   179
Maria's Birth Story   *184*
Lotus Birth   *186*

Water Birth   188
  Tips for Getting Ready   190

The Third Stage of Labour   **192**
  The Third Stage: Delivering the Placenta   192
  Care of the Cord   193
  Cord Stem Cell Collection   193
  Stem Cells: What Are They Used For?   194

Newborn Tests and Screening   **196**
  Heel Prick Test   196
  Vaccination   196
  Vitamin K   197
  Circumcision   197

Breast Is Not "Best" – It's Just Normal   **198**
  What's so Special about Breastmilk?   198
  Some Truths about Breastmilk   200
  Tips for Success   201
  Look at the Baby Not the Scale   204
  Breastfeeding in the Longer Term   205
  Breastfeeding Support   206
  Kangaroo Care   207
  Infant Massage   207

Taking Care of Yourself After the Birth   **209**
  Your Body   209
  Your Emotions   210
  Postnatal Depression   211
  Preventing and Coping with PND   212

**What Your Parents Never Warned You about
Becoming Parents**   **215**
  Why do Babies Cry?   215
  Helping Toddlers Adjust to a New Baby   219
  Tips to Prepare your Toddler   219
  Parenting Styles   220
  The Evolution of a Mother   221
  And Finally . . .   223

**Appendix A: Guide to Maternity Units in
Ireland**   **224**
  Spontaneous Onset of Labour   224
  Labour Induced   225
  Spontaneous Vaginal Birth   227
  Instrumental Birth (Vacuum/Forceps)   228
  Caesarean Birth   229
  Episotomy   230
  Initiated Breastfeeding within First Hour of Birth 232
  Exclusively Breastfeeding on Discharge from Hospital 233
  Statistics for Homebirth with Self-Employed
    Community Midwives for 2009   234

**Appendix B: Government Guidelines: What Are
Your Options?**   **237**
  Care Options   237
  Pregnancy and Employment Guidelines   240
  Maternity Leave   242
  Maternity Benefit   248

Glossary   249

Resources   255

Recommended Reading   259

Index   261

About the Author

Tracy Donegan is the Director of Doula Ireland, Founder of GentleBirth and mother of two gorgeous boys. Passionate about empowering parents to have the best birth possible, Tracy also runs the Irish chapter of the International Caesarean Awareness Network, a support group for parents affected by caesarean birth. Tracy's second book, *The Irish Caesarean and VBAC Guide* (Original Press, 2010), is available now.

Acknowledgements

Thank you to all of the mothers involved in the second edition of this book. Although many childbirth professionals provided assistance, the real experts are the mothers and families who are choosing to bring their babies into the world, calmly, gently and with confidence.

To my own family, Jack, Cooper and Philip for your unending patience and humour as Mammy worked on this second edition.

I am indebted to the following for advice, inspiration and permission to publish some of their insights: Ina May Gaskin, Dr. Michel Odent, Sheila Kitzinger, Andrea Robertson, Ethel Byrnes, Gail Tully, Laura Shanley, AIMS Ireland and Cuidiu. Thank you also to the people behind the following websites to reproduce and adapt some of their material: www.sarahjbuckley.com, www.AIMS-Ireland.com, www.Mothering.com; www.birthpsychology.com; www.DancingForBirth.com and the other websites and sources credited in the text.

To the Midwives of Ireland

"Courage doesn't always roar. Sometimes courage is the quiet
voice at the end of the day saying, 'I will try again tomorrow'."
– Mary Anne Radmacher

Introduction

Why This Book?

Why should you read this book? Simple really: if you are having a baby in Ireland, you want to know about Irish maternity care. Shelves in bookshops are straining under the weight of books on pregnancy and birth, but almost all written from a US or UK perspective. Irish women have told me again and again that they want a book written by an Irish woman for Irish women. So here it is!

Being pregnant is a wonderful experience for most of us. (Of course, we're all guilty of indulging in a little griping now and then!) But how can you really take the time to enjoy pregnancy when you have so many decisions to make? Plus, it seems like the closer the big day looms, the more decisions you have — and you're on a deadline that keeps moving! *The Irish Better Birth Book* answers the questions you have and more importantly those you never even thought to ask, so you can make the best choices for you and your baby.

We are bombarded with opinions and studies about pregnancy and birth. We hear reports on the news, we read about it online, we get tons of unsolicited advice from our friends and relatives. What or whom should we believe? How can we make sense of it all, especially when faced with important decisions that can have lasting effects on ourselves and our children? Years ago, the biggest decision you had to make was what colour to paint the baby's room! Now, it's "public or private?"; "home or hospital?"; "midwife or consultant?"; "epidural or natural?"; "kneeling or squatting?" . . . you get the picture.

So where do you even begin? Well, let's start with the star of the show: your new baby. There has always been a lot of focus on the mother's experience and how different choices can affect her.

It's only very recently that science has started to look at the baby's experience of pregnancy and birth. Once you bring your baby into the decision-making, then that mountain of choices you have to make becomes much more manageable. Now, unless you have an exceptionally gifted baby that can do Morse code on your organs (kicking your bladder for "yes" and your ribs for "no") it's quite difficult to get your baby's views on anything! So how do you know what is best for your baby? You will want to be sure that every choice you make is based on sound research (i.e. backed by science) so that any medical choice – whether it's antenatal testing, birth positions, drugs, etc. – is made on the basis of real medical indications. It should not just be something that is done routinely for everybody. Throughout the book, I have attempted to indicate in plain English what the latest and best research says about a particular option you have.

Fear-Free Birth

There are two kinds of realities: factual reality (supported by science) and perceived reality (your beliefs, and/or your caregiver's beliefs) It is a fact that in the western world around 80 to 90 per cent of mothers will have normal pregnancies and give birth between 37 and 42 weeks without any problems. But the perceived reality for many women is that birth is a disaster waiting to happen. It doesn't matter what science tells us if we believe otherwise. Our beliefs have been formed throughout our childhood and teenage years and won't just change overnight. Most mothers believe that our bodies are destined to fail and have forgotten the fact that we've been having babies for millions of years. It is a myth that birth became safer once it was moved to the hospital. Science tells us that, for low-risk pregnancies (most of you reading this book), home birth is in fact the better option – and yet our hospitals are still full every day of mothers with low-risk pregnancies. Facing our fears means we have to ask ourselves: Is this fear a factual reality (supported by science and best evidence) or is it my perception?

Another reason for writing this book is to dispel much of the fear and many of the myths that seem to surround pregnancy these days. When did pregnancy get to be such a worrying and fearful time? Whatever happened to blissfully happy mums-to-be? Our instant information age probably has a lot to do with it. You just have to log on to any pregnancy chat room or forum and instead of chatting with expectant mothers, you're bombarded with topics such as "stabbing pains", "c-section scar infection", "swollen fingers", "my baby is too small", "my baby is too big", "I'm anaemic", "I'm not anaemic" . . . No doubt you've heard that if you have morning sickness, then that "proves" that baby is doing fine – it's the "hormones" . . . but if you're one of those women who are lucky enough not to have morning sickness (or, as some call it, morning, noon and night sickness), then you worry yourself to death for a few weeks wishing you would throw up! How ridiculous is that?!

While I could blame the internet for all of this scary information, daytime TV doesn't exactly help. In these shows, we'll innocently follow a cheerful woman talking about her forthcoming "event" – and then cut to the birth where they say something like, "Will Claire and her baby survive? We'll find out right after this break!" Such suspense works fine for the X-Factor, but for a show about birth?! So, of course, we're all glued to our seats, thinking, "If it can happen to Claire, it could happen to me" when, in fact, most pregnancies are low risk. You've heard the horror stories from family and friends over the years. When was the last time you heard a positive birth story? Doctors themselves are also guilty of projecting their own beliefs or perceptions rather than the statistical realities.

So despite the "risky" tests, the possible perils of filling your car with petrol or eating mayonnaise with your ham sandwich, the recklessness of drinking a caffeinated beverage or having a sip of wine at a wedding, the odds are overwhelmingly in a pregnant woman's favour that, around 40 weeks or so from conception, one way or another and mostly regardless of what she has or hasn't done, the average pregnant woman will give birth and her baby will be just fine. Talk to women who have recently "passed over" to motherhood and they'll tell you that they wish they had spent a lot more time sleeping than worrying about whether or not they should have eaten that tuna sandwich for lunch. They'll also tell you to relax and enjoy your pregnancy (swollen ankles and all) because you only get one chance to carry your little bundle of joy this close to you, all to yourself, for the rest of her life and yours.

How to Use This Book

This book is intended as a guide to the experience of labour and childbirth. Much of what you read in these pages will differ from what you usually hear in hospital antenatal classes or read about in the mainstream pregnancy magazines. My hope is that after reading it, you may question some of your own beliefs about birth and maybe get a glimpse of how wonderful birth and becoming a new mum can be.

There is a huge amount of information available on pregnancy and birth. Sometimes, this can be truly bewildering. I have made use of some of the best available resources to bring to you the latest and best evidence on everything from how to make informed choices about the type of care you receive, to complementary therapies, to pain relief in labour. Look out for shaded boxes to guide you through these issues. And there are simple, practical tips that you can use to deal with everything from home birth to getting your baby into the best position for birth to breastfeeding. For these practical tips, just look out for the following little picture:

There is a glossary on pages 249–254 to explain some of the more unfamiliar terms (and some that you may be familiar with). In the text, I have highlighted terms that are explained in the glossary, usually on their first use, by writing them in bold print, and by this little picture in the margin:

Simple! If only figuring out your maternity benefit were as easy. But don't worry, we cover that in Appendix B, along with other government guidelines on rights and entitlements. And Appendix A provides information on hospital policies and statistics on some of the issues and choices discussed in the book, to help guide you towards the form of care that you feel suits you best.

As this is a book about birth I have only touched on pregnancy. Some great books on pregnancy are:

◊ *Pregnancy and Childbirth* by Sheila Kitzinger

◊ *Ina May's Guide to Childbirth* by Ina May Gaskin

◊ *Pregnancy, Childbirth and the Newborn* by Penny Simkin

◊ *Having a Baby Naturally* by Peggy O'Mara.

These and other books of interest are listed at the back of the book.

Throughout the book I have included actual birth stories to illustrate what a momentous event birth is in our lives, and how every birth is different. (I have changed names and some details to preserve privacy.) What will your birth story be? My hope is that your birth story will be one of excitement and empowerment – the excitement of those first labour twinges and the empowerment of being informed and confidently making the right choices for you and your baby.

In fact, I want to end this introduction with a highly unusual, but incredibly empowering birth story from the US – unusual in the sense that it shows that it is possible to have a fear-free, pain-free birth experience. Laura Shanley is the mother of four children, all born at home without the help of doctors or midwives. Laura's husband, David, caught their first baby and Laura herself caught the other three. Neither of them had been trained in midwifery or medicine. Today, the Shanleys teach other women their methods. Perhaps one day a birth story such as theirs will not be so unusual . . .

Do-It-Yourself Childbirth

By Laura Shanley

Prepare to be amazed: I had an unassisted conception. My husband and I closed the bedroom door, took off our clothes, and conceived a child without any help from anyone! David got an erection without drugs of any sort, and actually proceeded to impregnate me without consulting a manual or consultant.

Even more amazing is that I didn't have a conception coach! No one stood next to the bed shouting "Push! Push! Pant! Pant!" Somehow, I just knew what to do!

Are you shocked? Are you impressed? Probably not. This is because the majority of babies in the world have been safely conceived this way throughout all of eternity. So why are you amazed when I say that I also had an unassisted pregnancy and birth?

"Well," you say, "because conception is easy, but pregnancy and birth are not." I beg to differ. Pregnancy is a natural, healthy condition. It is not a disease. If a woman is physically and psychologically healthy, there is absolutely no need to measure her tummy, test her urine, or check her blood. Needles hurt because skin is not designed to be punctured.

Even if a woman isn't healthy, does she really need a "professional" to inform her of the fact? Are women totally incapable of determining the state of their own health? And suppose they aren't healthy. Can a "professional" actually make them well? Perhaps if they believe in the professional more than they believe in themselves. I believe I am my own best caregiver. I have much more faith in my own abilities than I've ever had in any doctor or midwife.

Childbirth – the word alone makes most people cringe. Instantly, one imagines a frightened, tearful woman lying in a hospital bed surrounded by masked men and women and perhaps a family member. Monitors are beeping and people are yelling "PUSH! PUSH!" as the poor woman struggles with all her might to expel her baby. Her forehead is sweating and periodically she cries, "I can't do this anymore!" Medical personnel assure her that she can – but if she can't, they will be more than happy to assist her with drugs, forceps, scissors and a knife, if necessary. Thank God for modern medicine. How did we ever survive without it?

The truth is, we did survive and can continue to survive, quite well in most cases, especially when it comes to giving birth. First, however, we must rid ourselves of the belief that childbirth is a painful, dangerous ordeal that must always be supervised and assisted by "skilled professionals". I chose to believe otherwise, and this is my story.

I first became interested in childbirth when I was about six years old. After listening to my mother's explanation of what actually happens in birth, however, my interest was short lived. "After they shave you, the doctor makes a little cut to make more room for the baby," she said. That's all I needed to hear. If there were to be any children in my future, someone else was going to have to give birth to them.

Changing Perceptions

As I grew older, movies and television helped fill in all the gory details. Obviously, I reasoned, pregnancy was a disease complete with vomiting, backaches, swollen ankles and strange cravings. If you survived it, you could look forward to hours or maybe days of excruciating labour pains, followed by weeks in the hospital. Motherhood was becoming increasingly unappealing.

My perception of childbirth changed, however, when at the age of 18 my husband-to-be, David, presented me with a copy of Grantly Dick-Read's *Childbirth Without Fear*. Dick-Read was an English physician who used chloroform to ease labour pains, as was the custom in the first half of the twentieth century. But one night, something happened that forever changed his perception of birth.

He went to the house of a poor countrywoman who was about to have a child. When he felt the birth was near, he offered her the chloroform, but the woman refused to take it. This was the first time he had ever seen a woman refuse it, and yet the woman remained perfectly calm and the baby was born easily. As he was leaving, he asked her why she had chosen to give birth without an anaesthetic and she replied, "It didn't hurt. It wasn't meant to, was it, doctor?"

Over the next few years, Dick-Read encountered other women who appeared to have little or no pain in childbirth. What, he wondered, could explain why some women suffered and others did not. He went on to study it extensively. He discovered that the women who suffered the most in childbirth were the ones who were most afraid.

Fear, he learned, has a profound effect on the body. When a person is in a state of fear, messages are sent to the body telling it to either fight the perceived danger or run away from it. Blood and oxygen instantly rush into the muscle structure, which in turn gives the body the power it needs to survive. Any organs that are not needed for either "fight or flight" are consequently drained of blood (and oxygen) so that it may be diverted elsewhere. This explains why people turn "white as a sheet" when they're afraid. The body assumes that the face is not in need of blood and oxygen as much as the legs, for instance, which when given the extra "fuel", enable the endangered person to run.

In addition to the face, blood is also drained from the brain, the digestive organs and the uterus. Dick-Read found that the uterus of a frightened woman in labour is literally white. Without the fuel it needs, the uterus cannot function correctly, nor can waste products be carried away. Therefore, labour hurts. The solution — eliminate the fear and you eliminate the pain.

Dick-Read's theories made sense to me. Maybe childbirth wouldn't be so bad after all, I thought. Less than two years later, David and I moved in together and I got the chance to see for myself.

In addition to *Childbirth Without Fear*, we had also been reading other books that dealt with how our beliefs create our reality. Little by little, we were beginning to create the life we desired. Why, we wondered, shouldn't we be able to create the birth we desired, as well? In November 1977, I conceived.

Every day I repeated my belief suggestions. "I believe in my ability to give birth safely and easily at home," I told myself. "I believe I'm not afraid, I believe I'm safe, I believe I'm innocent. I believe I'm deserving of a good birth." I examined every aspect of my consciousness, looking for any beliefs that might prevent me from having the kind of birth I desired. I also practised giving birth frequently in my dreams.

Consequently, I had almost none of the so-called symptoms of pregnancy. I vomited only one day, and that stopped when I realised I still had some fears about becoming a mother. "I'm not afraid of being a mother," I told myself, and I never vomited again.

I went into labour on the afternoon of 20 August 1978. The contractions weren't completely painless, but they weren't anything that I couldn't easily handle. Around midnight, David and I called up three of our friends who had asked to attend, along with a filmmaker who wanted to film the birth. Within a half an hour, everyone was there, and we proceeded to talk and laugh and generally enjoy ourselves. We didn't time contractions or check to see how dilated I was. We simply relaxed, had fun, and trusted that when the time was right, the baby would be born.

At about 1.30 am, my water bag broke and I reached down and felt the baby's face. I walked over to the bed, got on my hands and knees, and was about to turn over when I heard an inner voice say, "Don't turn over." I didn't, and a second later my beautiful baby boy, John, literally flew into David's hands. The birth had been a tremendous success. Fifteen months later, I conceived my second son, Willie, and also delivered him, feet first, at home into my own hands. Eighteen months after having Willie, I conceived my daughter, Joy.

This time I thought I might like to be alone for the birth. I had come to trust my body completely. On the morning of 17 November 1982, I went into labour. My sons were sleeping and David was at the campus library. I took a shower, got out my little bathtub, and got down on one foot and one knee, the position that felt right to me this time. When I felt her head crowning, I gave one push and she slipped gently into my hands. She looked right up at me and gave a little cry. The thought went through my mind that she was the most beautiful gift I had ever received.

After cutting the cord, wrapping her in a blanket and delivering the placenta into the bathtub, I went over to the couch to lie down. Soft bells and the sound of ocean waves filled my head. I felt positively blissful. An hour or two later, I got up and took a shower. Then Joy, John, Willie, a friend of mine and I all walked over to the campus to see David. The temperature was in the 70s and I felt as if I were floating on air. This, I thought, is how birth is supposed to be.

A Relaxed Birth

My last child, Michelle, was born on 5 April 1987. That morning I awoke feeling mild contractions. David was up reading the paper, but I decided not to tell him that I was in labour. As I lay in my bed, I breathed deeply and said belief suggestions. I told myself, "I'm moving out of the way and allowing my body to give birth." Suddenly I felt myself slip into a state of complete relaxation. I had absolute faith that the consciousness within me that knew how to grow my baby perfectly, also knew how to get my baby out. My job was simply to relax and allow it to happen.

An hour later, I decided to get up and take a bath. I walked across the hall, turned on the bath water and sat down on the toilet. As I looked between my legs, I saw my water bag beginning to protrude. It popped, I gave a little push, and my little girl slipped into my hands. "David," I called out, "will you come here a minute?"

David came down the hall and was amazed to see Michelle sitting on my lap, peacefully nursing. "You'd better find a scissors," I said, "and turn off the bath water, please."

My story is not unique. Throughout history, women have given birth successfully without medical assistance. In fact, the infant mortality rate in this country rose sharply after women began giving birth in hospitals. Even today, numerous studies show that for the majority of women, home birth is actually safer than hospital birth.

Childbirth is a natural process, which works best when it is interfered with least. Or, as Grantly Dick-Read writes, "If left alone in labour, the body of a woman produces most easily the baby that is not interfered with by its mother's mind or the assistant's hand."

Most childbirth "professionals", however, those whose income and self-esteem are dependent upon women turning themselves over to the "authorities" in labour, would have us believe otherwise. The truth is, with the proper beliefs, any woman can give birth easily, either by herself or in the company of a partner, friends or family. What better place to start believing in our own abilities than with the birth of a child?

© Laura Shanley. Adapted and reproduced with kind permission of the author. www.ucbirth.com

You're Pregnant! What Now?

There's a line – mother of God, there's a line!!

This is usually a time of great excitement and terror . . . and excitement . . . and more terror! I'm going to be somebody's mother – that thought scared me more than labour did. Every pregnancy is different, whether it's your first or fifth. It's normal to feel overwhelmed by the news that you're pregnant. You're about to start the job of a lifetime (and you may not have even applied for it). Even if this pregnancy is something you were planning, the realisation of actually being pregnant is like getting on a rollercoaster for the first time; once the ride starts, you're on it until the end. How much you enjoy the ride depends a lot on how you perceive the experience and who is there with you through the twists and turns, ups and downs. If you see pregnancy as being something to look forward to rather than a disruption to your life you'll enjoy the ride a lot more. Above all, keep in mind that pregnancy is temporary. You won't be pregnant forever (although it can feel like that towards the end).

If you think you are pregnant and those ten home pregnancy tests (just to be really really sure) are positive, the first step is usually to visit your GP, who will do some preliminary tests, such as taking your blood, weighing you, and will use the date of your last period to estimate the date the baby is due (this is a rough estimate, not an appointment; more on this later). You will then discuss your plans for antenatal care and what your expectations are for the birth. Your GP will then provide you with a "letter of referral" to the maternity hospital if that is where you plan to have your baby. (Not all hospitals insist on a letter of referral; you can just call the hospital directly.) If you're planning to have your baby at home, see the chapter on home birth. If you decide on having combined care you can save yourself a lot of time hang-

11

ing out in the hospital as most of your visits will be with your GP. (See Appendix B, pages 237–248 for more on combined care, public and private care, etc.)

The First Antenatal Visit

If you are going the hospital route, the first antenatal visit is always such an exciting one – and unfortunately it's usually a long one too. The visit can last about two hours (that may not even include waiting time). By contrast, you could blink and you'd miss your next visit, it'll be so quick, if your pregnancy is normal. Your first visit to hospital will probably be at any time from 12–20 weeks into the pregnancy. The purpose of this visit is to get a full picture of your health and the health of your baby. You can expect to speak to a **midwife**, who will ask a range of background questions about your health and medical history. This will also be an opportunity for you to ask about your care and the range of services that are available to you. You will be asked for a urine sample (get used to peeing in a cup – you'll have it down to a fine art by the time your baby is born), will have your blood pressure taken and will have some blood tests. In some hospitals you may have an **ultrasound** scan on your first visit; at others you will have this scan at around 20 weeks.

A general external physical examination will probably be carried out during your antenatal visit and usually includes the following:

◊ Abdomen, to determine the size of your growing baby.

◊ Hands and legs, to check for varicose veins or swelling. Excessive swelling later on in your pregnancy may be a warning of **pre-eclampsia** (pregnancy-induced high blood pressure).

◊ Heart and lungs, to make sure your general health is good.

◊ Weight, which may be assessed together with results from other tests to detect any potential complications. This is optional – if you don't want to be weighed at each visit you can decline this. However, any sudden weight gain or swelling should be reported to your doctor.

At each subsequent antenatal visit, you will provide a urine sample, your blood pressure will be checked, and you may be weighed. If you have any questions at any of these visits – ask them! The only stupid question is the one you don't ask. If you're like me, you might want to write down a few questions as you think of them before each visit – just so you don't look like a rabbit caught in the headlights when your doctor asks, "Any questions?"

Antenatal Classes

When our second child was on the way, my wife and I attended an antenatal class aimed at couples that had already had at least one child. The instructor raised the issue of breaking the news to the older child. It went like this: "Some parents," she said, "tell the older child, 'We love you so much we decided to bring another child into this family.' But think about that. Ladies, what if your husband came home one day and said, 'Honey, I love you so much I decided to bring home another wife.'" One of the women spoke up immediately. "Does she cook?"

Antenatal classes in Ireland provide you with information about pregnancy, labour and delivery, and baby care. Understanding the basic physiology of birth is important for all mothers (although most of us already know that the stork doesn't actually bring the baby). However, surprisingly, the importance of the hormone balance for an easy birth is rarely discussed (see pages 84–86). Ironically, most antenatal classes focus on coping strategies for the side effects (severe pain and longer labours) that come from disturbing this delicate balance of hormones.

The classes will also allow you to discuss any concerns you might have with other expectant parents. When everyone at work rolls their eyes when you mention swollen ankles again or, God forbid, the dreaded piles, it's such a treat to have so many sympathisers at the antenatal classes – safety in numbers. Many antenatal classes focus purely on labour and delivery, but others include practical advice on how to care for your baby and adjust to parenthood.

Antenatal classes are provided by hospitals and independent educators such as Cuidiu (The Irish Childbirth Trust), who are not associated with any particular hospital. They fill up quickly so book your place early. Classes are generally offered for first-time mothers alone or for couples. You will probably attend antenatal classes from about 20 to 30 weeks. Some hospitals are happy to have fathers come along to just one or two of the classes (much to the delight of most dads). Some hospitals also provide classes for couples with special needs and refresher classes for couples having their second baby. Classes are generally held over six to eight sessions (there are also intensive one day or weekend courses) and topics covered may include:

◊ Looking after your health during pregnancy

◊ Growth and development of the baby during pregnancy

◊ What to expect when you go into labour

◊ Options for labour and delivery

◊ Pain relief during labour

◊ Breastfeeding

◊ Physical care of your baby

◊ Returning to work/childcare arrangements.

Most antenatal classes are held by your local public maternity hospital and are free of charge. There may be benefits to taking antenatal classes run by independent practitioners as you'll get a good overview of the routine procedures and policies in many hospitals and not just the one you are attending. However, these are not free.

Dumb Excuses Not to Take Antenatal Classes

By Patricia Newton

I think I already know enough between watching television birthing shows and reading

In the eyes of some women, watching television birthing shows regularly is equal to true education. What you may not realise, however, is that what is shown as routine procedures on any particular episode is not necessarily what might occur routinely in the hospital where you will be giving birth. Common interventions vary widely from region to region, and from one caregiver to another.

In addition, because most of these shows are condensed to fit into 30 minutes (including commercials!), you do not see everything that led up to a particular point in any labour. For example, if a woman's labour stalls or stops, there are many reasons why this could happen. There are also several things the woman could try to help speed her labour or get it started again before medical interventions are needed. However, these informative issues are seldom shown or discussed in these shows.

What would be more helpful to you would be to enrol in a good childbirth education class, taught by a professional who is familiar with the common birthing practices in your area. In such a class you would learn the pros and cons of these procedures and be encouraged to discuss any concerns you may have with your own care provider.

As for reading, there are many excellent books available for the pregnant woman. Some of them are *Ina May's Guide to Childbirth* by Ina May Gaskin; *Gentle Birth Choices* by Barbara Harper; *Pregnancy, Childbirth and the Newborn* by Penny Simkin, Janet Whalley and Ann Keppler; and *Mind Over Labour* by Carl Jones.

Mums who have previously given birth say you forget everything you heard in class once that first contraction hits

Any childbirth education class worth your time will teach you many tools you can use during the stages of labour. Some of these tools are deep relaxation, massage, faith, vocalisation, aromatherapy, changing positions, and affirmations. There are many others to learn about as well.

However, being given tools and actually practicing them are two very different things. You might learn of breathing techniques or labouring positions in class, but if you decide not to practise any of the important tools at home, chances are you won't be ready to use them to your advantage once labour begins.

If you are serious about preparing for labour, you will become very familiar with the many things you can do to cope with contractions, shorten your labour and reduce your pain. And if you become familiar with them during pregnancy, you will know how to use them properly during your labour.

On the other hand, if you are not dedicated to practising and preparing, you just might not have a clue how to deal with contractions. But is that the fault of the antenatal teacher?

The nurses are there to help you get through labour

Midwives would love to be able to give you one-to-one continuous support during your labour, but the many demands of their job may not allow them to do this. They are also required to monitor, chart, keep doctors informed of the status of their patients and administer medications. And if they have more than one patient in labour, they have to take care of that patient as well. In addition, midwives have breaks from their shift and there comes a time when their shift ends. Which means they leave and a different midwife is assigned to you.

Although midwives are likely to help you work through contractions for short periods of time, they may not be able to stay beside you and witness every contraction you face. In most cases, they are not someone with whom you already have a bond. Your midwife is usually someone you don't know well, or someone you've never even seen before.

So, skipping the childbirth education class and planning on having a midwife provide continuous labour support for you may not be a realistic plan.

> *I'd rather spend the money on something for the baby*
>
> Yes, independent childbirth education classes do cost money. But spending your money on something for your baby instead of a class that can truly help you have a shorter, easier and safer labour with an end result of a healthier baby comes down to one thing: a matter of priority.
>
> Only you can decide what you think is more important.
>
> Along with pregnancy comes responsibility. Responsible parents make decisions during pregnancy in the best interest of their child. This begins with choosing a medical care provider who is right for them and attending an informative, empowering childbirth education class.
>
> © *Patricia Newton, a leading childbirth educator, lactation educator and doula (www.proudpregnancies.com)*

Ultrasound Scans

Your first ultrasound may well be the moment when everything becomes real. You knew you were pregnant, but now you get to see the little person who is turning your world upside down, and you haven't had the pleasure of meeting them yet. It's an emotional moment for many parents. The first scan is usually offered to pregnant women at around 12–14 weeks (sometimes referred to as your early "dating" or "booking" scan). This is when your caregiver will give you your **EDD** (your guess date); early scans are usually more accurate. In certain circumstances, for example, if there are any particular risks or problems, you may be able to have earlier or later scans if necessary.

How Do They Work?

An ultrasound scan transmits silent sound waves through your body tissues to create an image of your baby in your womb, which you and your partner will be able to see on a screen.

Before having your scan, you'll sometimes be asked to drink plenty of fluid and not to empty your bladder; if your bladder is full, it then pushes up against your womb to give a better view of your baby. When you are lying down, your stomach will be covered with a gel (it's usually freezing; would it kill them to heat it up?) and a handheld transducer will be moved in various directions over your skin to allow you to see your baby inside your womb. While the scan is being carried out, the operator will usually explain what she/he is looking at, and you may be given a black-and-white printout of the picture to take home.

Ultrasound scans can also be carried out using a vaginal probe (usually in early pregnancy). This is not very common in Ireland and is more likely to be used if you've had bleeding early on and suspect a miscarriage.

Why Are They Done?

Ultrasound scans don't take long to complete and are used for various reasons, although their main purpose is to check:

◊ How many babies you are carrying

◊ How far along in pregnancy you are

◊ If your baby is developing normally and to monitor its growth.

Not only can ultrasound scans measure your baby's size and shape, to give a better idea of age and date of delivery, but they can also:

◊ Show the exact position of your baby and the **placenta**

◊ Assess bleeding in early pregnancy

◊ Identify growth problems, especially of the head or spine, check the levels of **amniotic fluid** and blood flow through the **umbilical cord**.

◊ Be used to guide certain diagnostic tests or operations that may have to be undertaken on your baby in the womb.

Are They Safe?

There continues to be some debate around the safety of ultrasounds and the effects on the unborn baby, although most doctors consider them safe. There was a time when x-rays were considered safe for pregnant women. Ultrasounds have never conclusively been proven to be harmful, but they have also never conclusively been proven to be 100 per cent safe.

What If There's a Problem?

Although getting a scan is usually an exciting time for some parents, the news is not always good. Here are some questions to ask if your scan shows a problem:

1. What exactly is the problem?

2. How serious is the problem?

3. What will it mean for my baby if he/she is born with this problem?

4. Are you quite sure about what the scan is showing?

5. Is there a better scanner in this or another hospital, which could give a more detailed picture?

6. What are my options now?

7. How quickly do I have to make up my mind about what to do?

8. Can you provide me with support group information for this particular diagnosis?

Making the Best Choices for You and Your Baby

What about My Baby?

There has been a lot of focus on the mother's experience of birth and how different choices can affect her. What about the baby? How are our babies affected by the choices we make as expectant mothers?

Most of us now know that our unborn baby is an aware, reacting human being who, from about the sixth month on, leads an active emotional life. Your baby can hear, taste, experience and, on a primitive level, learn in utero. (But before you start playing French tapes to your bump, at this point the only thing your baby needs to know is how much he is wanted.) Much research suggests that what a child feels and perceives begins shaping his attitudes and expectations about himself and can actually have a great effect on his personality development in later life.

There have been significant advances in the study of how our babies are affected by our actions and feelings before and during birth. In an interesting piece of research several years ago Dr Michael Lieberman showed that an unborn child grows emotionally agitated (measured by his heart rate) each time his mother thinks of having a cigarette. Just the idea of having a cigarette is enough to upset the baby. Of course, the baby has no way of knowing his mother is smoking or thinking about it but his brain is sophisticated enough to associate the experience of her smoking with the unpleasant sensation it produces in him. It puts him in a constant state of uncertainty and fear. He just never knows when the unpleasant sensation will happen again. (What better reason to give up cigarettes!)

After months of floating peacefully, birth is the first prolonged emotional and physical shock your baby undergoes – and he never quite forgets it. **Oxytocin**, a hormone that our body produces in labour, has an amnesic affect (causes you to forget). We know that birth memories exist and can be retrieved with a qualified therapist. Dr David B. Cheek has focused his attention specifically on birth memories and his work is very significant. Through hypnosis, Dr Cheek has been able to retrieve birth memories about specific incidents which only he would be aware of, such as the angle of the baby's head when it descends. If a child can remember something as miniscule as how his head was turned at birth, what about those children who have traumatic births – emergency **caesarean section, forceps, vacuum**? How do these first experiences of life outside the womb affect their personalities? Similarly, how would a gentle birth experience affect him?

As mothers, all of our emotions are experienced by our babies. You are all-important to your developing unborn child. You are your infant's universe. What a huge responsibility! Although your baby doesn't yet have the vocabulary to understand what is being said around him, he feels stress when mum is stressed and feels happy when mum is happy. Isn't it time we put as much thought into our mental well-being as we do with our physical self?

Take a Baby Bonding Break Today!

You can send messages to your unborn child by the emotions you feel. The best way to send the message is by taking several baby breaks a day. First, find some music that you enjoy and that makes you feel good. Listen to music that gives you the feeling of peace, joy and love. It might be an old song that brings back happy memories or just the sound of the waves on the beach. (Get those endorphins going!) Play it so your unborn baby can hear it (don't use earphones) and then relax by taking several deep breaths while sitting or lying in a restful position. Fill your senses with a peaceful scene like a mountain lake or beach. Be sure to use all of your senses. See the ocean, hear the waves, feel the sand and sun, smell the salt air.

This may take some practice, but after several attempts you will start feeling your own body's response to the mental picture. That's when you know you are sending a message to your baby. I suggest you take a 20-minute baby bonding break once or twice a day

21

— more if you're really feeling stressed. This practice has many benefits to you and to your unborn child. It will programme your child's emotional temperament and give him/her the expectation of peace and love in his or her universe after birth. Do it standing at the bus stop, or sitting in traffic — make it something easy to incorporate into what is no doubt an already busy life.

Many antenatal yoga classes include mother/baby bonding sessions, which is a wonderful way to get to know your baby before birth. We desperately need antenatal care that puts as much emphasis on the mother and child's emotional needs as it does on the physical ones.

Being aware of your unborn child's consciousness and awareness should make the birth planning process easier. When you understand that every choice you make can have a positive or negative effect on your baby, making the right decision gets a whole lot easier.

© *Frederick Wirth MD. Adapted and reproduced with kind permission from* Prenatal Parenting: The Complete Psychological and Spiritual Guide to Loving Your Unborn Child

Each pregnancy and each birth is different. The following are two very different birth stories, the first of a number you will find in this book. (Please note that all names and some details of births have been changed for all birth stories in this book.)

Therese's Birth Story

My labour started on a Monday but at that stage I wasn't aware, as a first-time mum, that I was even in labour! I wasn't due for another two days; surely it couldn't be starting now! I had attended all of my antenatal classes, had got tips on what a Braxton Hicks was all about but still didn't know I was actually having a contraction on this Monday afternoon! I was bent over with pain and told myself that it was something I ate. I sat back down to watch TV and everything went back to normal.

On Tuesday morning I got up, had a shower and felt great. I went shopping and did all the normal things a girl does to prepare for the birth of her baby. I went crazy washing clothes that didn't need washing, dusted the house from top to bottom and cooked chicken that was already cooked! I went back to watching television, feet up . . . I felt just fine. Later that evening I felt completely exhausted and went to bed early about 8.00 pm. I kept wondering if I was going to deliver my baby on the expected due day, or would it be overdue by two weeks. I couldn't get comfortable and kept feeling a niggling pain all over my tummy. I was getting excited and thought "there's something going on"! I just couldn't relax and kept getting up to walk around.

I rang my sister Mary at about 10.00 pm to discuss it with her, as she had two children. She said this was the start of labour and I was even more excited. She told me to take a shower and time the contractions. At this stage they were coming every 30 minutes and bearable.

Mary said to stay at home until at least midnight and then she would collect me. I had already had a shower earlier that day and while having a second one my mother shouted up to me, "Why are you having another shower when you already had one this morning, you will wash yourself down the drain!" I didn't want to alarm her so I told her I was just trying to cool myself down. At about 11.20 pm Mary arrived; my mother asked what she was doing up at the house at that hour of the night. My sister replied "It's time!" That's when my mother started to panic!

At 11.30 pm the contractions were coming full force and I was doing my breathing techniques, which helped a great deal. We headed into the Rotunda Hospital and made it for 12.05 am. In the admissions room was told I was 5cm dilated and was asked if I wanted the epidural and I said "Yes!" We took the lift up to the delivery suite, where I met with my midwife who was lovely and so relaxed. I was so excited I couldn't wait to give birth. I already knew that my obstetrician was away for that bank holiday weekend, but surprised me by turning up just after I had given birth.

I got the epidural, which was scary to say the least. I didn't go for the gas or pethidine or anything else. It took over an hour to get the epidural needle, which quickly set in. When it did kick in, I felt great!

23

I was relaxed and the midwife asked me if I knew whether I was having a boy or a girl and I told her a girl as people had been telling me that I had "it all in the back and sides" and every time I went to a clothes shop for kids I was drawn to the pink section, so I had convinced myself that I was having a girl! I was chatting away when the midwife told me to start pushing; and push I did. A very short time later, at 3.30 am, I delivered a beautiful baby boy! I was very surprised but ecstatic when I realised it was a boy!

I have to say the whole experience of pregnancy and childbirth was surprising and enjoyable. I sailed through it. I was so absolutely overjoyed with the birth experience that I would have had another baby there and then! The staff were excellent and I even got a private room to share with my beautiful son alone! It was the happiest day of my life and I will treasure that for the rest of my life.

◇◇◇

◇◇◇

Ann's Birth Story

My son Jake was born at 10 am on a Saturday, three days before his due date. Being a first timer, I was quite idealistic about birth and certain I could cope with whatever came my way. I had read several books and attended both an active birth class and a regular antenatal class. Although I wanted to keep an open mind, I was hoping for a natural birth and made out a birth plan (amended several times) to reflect this.

It started off pretty well. A couple of days before the birth I felt very restless and had huge surges of energy. Everyone told me I would go overdue on my first, so I was surprised to feel a few funny little twinges on the Wednesday night. I thought they were kind of painful at the time (how naïve in retrospect!) but decided I was constipated as I couldn't believe it was anything else.

By Thursday evening, they started feeling a little stronger. These were achy cramps in my belly that definitely didn't feel normal. I was excited and nervous but unwilling to think this could be labour on the way, as I had so expected to go overdue.

My husband Tony had just bought a car that week and was learning how to drive. We expected to have a few weeks so he could practise the route to the hospital. We went for a practice drive that evening but all the stopping and starting was increasing the pain. It was completely manageable, however, and we put it down to maybe strong Braxton-Hicks. I had a glass of wine and a bath to relax me, but I was beginning to get pretty hyper now. I took advantage of this time and got plenty of massages and rolled around on my birthing ball.

In retrospect, I probably overdosed on active birth aids! I was hopping in and out of clary sage baths, trying various relaxation techniques, burning oils and pacing around the house all night. Needless to say, I was pretty exhausted by Friday morning. I hadn't slept and was starting to get very bored of amusing myself with aromatherapy and music while Tony slept soundly.

I had a "show" around 7.00 am and rang the hospital. The midwife on reception sounded quite blasé and told me to come in when contractions were three minutes apart. They were now about five to ten minutes apart but kept stopping and starting. I really wanted to wait at home as long as possible, so I went for a long walk with Tony, stopping every few minutes to bend into the contraction. It was all very weird and strangely enjoyable, just the two of us pretending to do normal things but with the anticipation of what lay ahead.

By nine that evening I felt I needed to get to the hospital. I'd had a bath and the pain really stepped up afterwards. I felt a bit sick and disorientated and was conscious of the shaky drive ahead. Tony got highly excited at my disorientated state and went to look it up in the books. "You're strange and confused. The books say you could be in transition!"

It couldn't be that quick, I thought. But the pain was very bad! We grabbed the bag and bundled into the car, convinced I was well on the way.

Neither of us will ever forget that drive. Tony's hands gripped the wheel until his knuckles were pure white. We drove through the city centre at 10.00 pm on a Friday, behind ambulances, police cars and pedestrians milling around. Tony missed the turn for the hospital three times and we went around in circles as he cursed and I kept quiet, breathing steadily through each pain.

We finally arrived in one piece. We were met by the midwife on duty. She berated me mildly for not coming in earlier and whisked me off to the examination room. Everything was done quickly and quietly. I think I may have been the only woman in labour there on a Friday night!

Tony was sent off to sign admittance forms and other documents that he admitted later to not really reading properly. I was swiftly hooked up to monitors and had an internal exam. I'd been dreading this but it was actually OK, not painful at all, just a little uncomfortable. I was convinced I would be well dilated; how disappointing to hear I was only 4 cm!

We were brought into a small little room with a bed, birthing ball and shower. It was dark and clinical and I suddenly felt really down and upset. Another long night stretched ahead and I didn't feel so in control anymore. Here in the hospital, I was just another woman in labour, to be dealt with quickly and professionally. All my breathing and labour techniques felt totally wrong here and I couldn't help wishing I'd stayed at home.

My consultant was away and had failed to deliver my birth plan to the midwives as he had promised. I had brought a copy with me and handed it over, a little shamefacedly I must admit.

The doctor on call took a look at my plan and said he fully supported my wish to birth without intervention. There was a proviso, however: I needed to get to 6 cm in the next three to four hours.

Talk about pressure! I was suddenly in a race, desperate to prove my competent cervix and superior labour ability to all these people. I thought with growing resentment of all those classes and books, describing contractions as "uncomfortable" and pain as "positive"; friends with children hiding their mirth as I earnestly outlined my high pain threshold and desire for a natural birth.

But I still felt that I could do this and that Tony and I would manage on our own. I drank tea and ate toast, managing each contraction pretty well and chatting with Tony. In the back of my mind I was worried that time was going slowly. I was dying for something to happen.

After another internal, I was told I wasn't dilating. We discussed breaking my waters; I agreed as I wanted things to speed up. I felt it made sense but the pain was horrible. The procedure was quick but felt nasty and invasive. After that, the contractions came very fast.

I walked around, did some yoga and breathed through each contraction. Waves of immense pain were coming closer and now it was impossible to focus on anything else. I knew it was bad when I wasn't able to drink juice or touch any of my high glucose snacks. I didn't want to be on all fours, on the birthing ball or have Tony near me.

Massages didn't work any more and I was getting desperate to find something to distract me. Part of me wished to be offered pain relief but I'd asked not to be offered it in my birth plan and was too stubborn to request it! However, I still felt I could just about control the pain by greeting it and breathing into it. I sat on the floor for ages and just meditated as best I could. I remember visualising the contractions: sometimes they were waves of white light building up from the pelvis right through my insides; sometimes I was climbing a hill and peaking and descending. It was all so long, sickening and exhausting.

I didn't move or disturb the rhythm as the midwife and Tony sat silently with me and watched. I was determined not to cry or groan as I feared that I would descend into panic if I did. I was so quiet that the midwife told me it was hard to believe a woman was in labour. She tried to encourage me but I really needed a new diversion now, something else to help me.

I was monitored and examined again and getting pretty impatient with all these procedures! The internal showed I had only moved 1 cm in the last few hours. I was 5 cm and completely demoralised.

The baby's heartbeat wasn't picking up too well anymore on the monitor. The doctor came in and examined me. He said the baby's head seemed quite small and that he was in the posterior position. He was worried about the heartbeat and, although he understood I didn't want a C-section, it might be necessary. I was getting close to not caring by then.

I was knackered and nauseous. I couldn't even drink water and I was really scared of the pain getting even worse – which the doctor assured me it would.

I took a shower and the hot water helped a little but I was getting confused and angry. I wanted someone to tell me what to do, or just to tell me I could do this, that I was managing. I had lost faith in my ability to do this. I was terrified and I wanted to go home!

The heart rate was still not picking up too well after contractions. The doctor suggested putting in a syntocinon drip to speed things up. He added that I'd find this very painful and would need an epidural as the contractions would be a lot worse. He added that a C-section was looking more and more likely if we didn't move fast to speed things up. I still felt I might manage it but I didn't know how much longer they would let me go on without a dreaded C-section. Plus the prospect of pain relief suddenly sounded like heaven.

Another hour passed before the anaesthetist arrived. I hadn't realised how high on natural endorphins I was until they hooked me up and turned on the drugs. As pain relief gradually flooded my body I felt all the adrenaline leave with a "whoosh".

All the voices and images in my head left suddenly and I lay on the delivery table, being turned and prodded, hooked up to all sorts of monitors, feeling a mixture of relief, shame and depression.

Having no pain was amazing and the awful fatigue and sickness left my body. But I felt I could have kept going, that I had "given in" somehow. I was also lost without my need to breathe and meditate. Tony went off for breakfast and I was alone with a new midwife on duty and an uninterested doctor. I lay there feeling sorry for myself, refusing to sleep.

As it turned out, I only had to wait an hour in that state. I was checked again and the syntocinon drip had worked its magic – I was 7 cm by now.

But the baby's heart rate was dropping and not recovering very well. The doctor told me again that a C-section might be necessary but we'd "try some pushing" first . . .

All this happened so fast. Tony said later he came back from breakfast and there I was on the table, legs akimbo and held up by midwives, starting to push. I delivered myself into their hands. This was the real deal — when it really happens. I don't think I can ever remember living so intensely in the moment as when I pushed. I visualised the rectum and held my breath as I bore down and used every ounce of my strength.

And they cheered me on, told me I was doing great — all the things I had dreaded. Even worse, I found myself somehow with my legs in stirrups — exactly what I had set out to avoid. I had pictured myself elegantly squatting and delivering the baby with a few quick pushes!

But it didn't matter right now. I was too caught up really participating again, now more than ever — and I liked it once I understood what I was doing. I breathed and pushed with incredible strength for 30 minutes and my son slithered out with one last almighty push.

And then this tiny, scared little creature plopped onto my tummy. His eyes were wide open and he looked straight up at me. I looked at him in astonishment and everything else ceased to exist for a moment.

I'm sure I cried but it's all a bit of a blur after that. I was unable to grasp it was all over and he was here. The team around me moved with ruthless efficiency, cleaning up the mess; the doctor chatted away as he gave me some stitches and Jake was whisked off to be put in an incubator as he was so small — only 4lbs 10oz.

I was given some tea and toast which tasted amazing and Tony and I were left alone for a while. We could hardly string words together; we were both shell shocked. I felt wired but also pretty confused. I wanted to relive every moment of the birth again and again and talk about every detail.

Jake was kept in the Special Care Unit for a week. In the days that followed I discovered that my placenta had most likely stopped functioning, which explained why he was so small. He had shown up as about 6lbs on the last scan two weeks before the birth, so had most likely lost weight in the womb. I never found out for sure what happened or whether it could have been avoided.

I can't say that birth was a joyous experience for me; the whole experience was overwhelming and it took me a while to get over it. While I am glad that I did arm myself with knowledge and a good birth plan, I know now that these can only take you so far. It's hard not to be a little idealistic your first time round and wish for a wonderful labour. My labour may not have been easy, but it had its wonderful moments!

Evidence-Based Care

There's a new catchphrase in medicine: **"evidence-based care"**. Evidence-based maternity care involves using the best research about the safety and effectiveness of specific tests, treatments and other interventions to help guide maternity care decisions. In a nutshell, evidence-based medicine is care based on the recommendations of the highest quality research available. To take a simple example, outside the area of maternity: suppose your sister falls and twists her ankle badly. Her doctor would follow guidelines specific to your sister's situation: after an examination, if all the signs point to there being a break, he would recommend an x-ray. Clinical recommendations drawn up following randomised controlled studies (the gold standard of research) show that the best course of action in this case is to confirm that there is a broken bone by taking an x-ray. This would be the practice of evidence-based medicine. Of course, the doctor could also have just sent your sister home with a set of crutches and a pressure bandage and told her to stay off her foot for a few days because, in his opinion, there are no bones broken. This would not be evidence-based medicine.

All maternity care needs to reflect "best practice" principles and be evidence-based. Telling you that your shoe size or your height will affect your chances of a successful vaginal birth would not be evidence-based care. Unfortunately, it seems that obstetrics takes a lot longer to follow evidence-based practices than most other areas of medicine. A good example of non-evidence-based policies often seen in Irish hospitals is the restriction of food and water to labouring mothers – more on this later.

The following piece sheds some international light on how Ireland's maternity system has developed. The author, Marsden Wagner, MD, is a perinatologist and perinatal epidemiologist from California and an outspoken supporter of midwifery. He was director of Women's and Children's Health in the World Health Organisation for 15 years.

Fish Can't See Water

By Marsden Wagner

Humanising birth means understanding that the woman giving birth is a human being, not a machine and not just a container for making babies. Showing women – half of all people – that they are inferior and inadequate by taking away their power to give birth is a tragedy for all society. On the other hand, respecting the woman as an important and valuable human being and making certain that the woman's experience while giving birth is fulfilling and empowering is not just a nice extra; it is absolutely essential as it makes the woman strong and therefore makes society strong.

But we do not have humanised birth in many places today. Why? Because fish can't see the water they swim in. Birth attendants, be they doctors, midwives or nurses, who have experienced only hospital-based, high interventionist, medicalised birth cannot see the profound effect their interventions are having on the birth.

These hospital birth attendants have no idea what a birth looks like without all the interventions, a birth which is not dehumanised. This widespread inability to know what normal, humanised birth is has been summarised by the WHO:

"By medicalising birth, i.e. separating a woman from her own environment and surrounding her with strange people using strange machines to do strange things to her in an effort to assist her, the woman's state of mind and body is so altered that her way of carrying through this intimate act must also be altered and the state of the baby born must equally be altered. The result is that it is no longer possible to know what births would have been like before these manipulations. Most health care providers no longer know what 'non-medicalised' birth is. The entire modern obstetric and neonatological literature is essentially based on observations of 'medicalised' birth." (World Health Organisation).

Why is medicalised birth necessarily dehumanising? In medicalised birth the doctor is always in control while the key element in humanised birth is the woman in control of her own birthing and whatever happens to her.

There is an expectation that there are guarantees of perfect outcomes with childbirth. **Obstetricians** are trained to think that "doing something is better than doing nothing" since the introduction of a high-tech approach to birth. It has lulled women and health professionals alike into a false sense of security that by providing the very best of appropriate care we can always avoid an unexpected outcome.

Although obstetric care is slowly becoming more evidence-based, there is a tendency not to evaluate routine interventions for their subtle and/or long-term risks. Another reason for the gap between evidence and practice is the excuses often given by consultants for why they reject evidence in their medical practice. These excuses include: the evidence is out of date; collecting evidence is too slow and prevents progress; they use clinical judgement and their opinion and experience; using anecdotal "horror stories" to try to prove the need for an intervention which the evidence has found unnecessary; quoting evidence which is of poor and/or inadequate quality; "trust me, I am a doctor".

In addition to these excuses, in maternity care common excuses include: our women have smaller pelvises (no evidence). Obstetricians tend to blind faith in technology and the mantra: technology = progress = modern. The other side of the coin is the lack of faith in nature, best expressed by a Canadian obstetrician: "Nature is a bad obstetrician."

Doctors replaced midwives for low-risk births, then science proved midwives safer. Hospital replaced home for low-risk birth, then science proved home as safe with far less unnecessary intervention. Hospital staff replaced family as birth support, then science proved birth safer if family present. Lying on your back replaced vertical birth positions, and then science proved vertical positions safer. Newborn examinations away from mothers in the first 20 minutes replaced leaving babies with mothers, then science proved the necessity for maternal attachment during this time. Man-made milk replaced woman-made milk, then science proved breastmilk superior. The central nursery replaced the mother, then science proved rooming-in superior. The incubator replaced the mother's body for care of low-weight newborns, then science proved the kangaroo method better in many cases.

© *Marsden Wagner. Adapted and reproduced with kind permission.*

So what does all this mean to you? Well, if your consultant or midwife routinely does **episiotomies**; recommends withholding food during labour; insists that you birth on the bed; automatically recommends c-section for a **breech**, **posterior** or even just a big baby without offering other options . . . they are not practising evidence-based care. You can choose to stay with this consultant or find one that shares the same philosophy on birth as you do.

The following article from a great resource, MaternityWise.org (The Maternity Center Association) explains the importance of making informed choices in your care.

Informed Decision Making, Informed Consent and Informed Refusal

By the Maternity Center Association

You are responsible for making informed decisions, and you have the legal right to give "informed consent" or "informed refusal".

Why is my involvement in maternity care decisions important?

As a pregnant woman, you have the opportunity and responsibility to make many important decisions about your care during pregnancy, birth and the time after birth. The decisions you make and the maternity care you receive can have lasting effects on the health and well-being of your baby, yourself and your family.

It is always important to understand whether there is a good rationale for any procedure, drug, test or treatment that is being given or offered to you. In many care settings, certain practices are used freely and even routinely, whether or not the mother or baby has shown a clear need. Although these practices may be of value to women or babies in certain situations, they may be unnecessary for most. They may be disruptive, be uncomfortable, cause more serious side effects and lead to the use of other interventions. For these reasons, interventions should not be used routinely or unnecessarily.

What does "making informed decisions" about maternity care mean?

Making informed decisions means learning and thinking about the best information available on maternity care, and then deciding what's right for you. Key questions for you to consider are:

◊   What are the possible choices?

◊   What does the best available research tell us about the safety and effectiveness of each of these choices?

◊   What are my needs and preferences and those of other family members?

◊   What choices are available and supported in my care setting?

◊   If I want an option that will not or may not be available to me, would I consider switching to a care setting or caregiver that does offer my preferred care?

Whenever possible, it is important to weigh this information well before you need to decide. This will help ensure that you can get answers to all of your questions and have access to the kind of care that is right for you.

How can I find the best evidence about safe and effective maternity care?

Dedicated health professionals also struggle to keep up with the vast amount of information relating to their practice and to know how to provide the best care.

Archie Cochrane, originator of the Cochrane Collaboration (a wonderful tool for researching evidence-based medicine) wondered which bits of medicine deserved the gold medal for being the most scientifically based and which deserved the wooden spoon for being the least scientific. . . . eventually he decided that it was the obstetricians that deserved the wooden spoon for being the least scientific doctors on the planet.

Fortunately, the evidence-based health care movement can help consumers and professionals alike sort out these complex matters.

What can I do to help ensure that the care that I receive during labour and birth will be best for me and my baby?

Your choice of caregiver and choice of birth setting (home or hospital) can have a major impact on the care that you receive during labour and birth. You may need to explore many possibilities to find a caregiver and birth setting that offer care consistent with the best evidence and with your needs and preferences.

It's not possible to know ahead of time exactly what your birth experience will be like. Being as informed as possible in advance will help you deal wisely with any new decisions that may arise at the time. It is important to learn about your options, get answers to your questions and think about your preferences well before labour begins. Be sure your partner, if you have one, is also aware of your wishes and is prepared to speak on your behalf if the need arises.

What does it mean to give "informed consent"?

Informed consent is a process to help you decide what will and will not be done to you and your body. In the case of maternity care, informed consent also gives you the authority to decide about care that affects your baby. The purpose of informed consent is to respect your right to self-determination. It empowers you with the authority to decide what options are in the best interest of you and your baby. Your rights to autonomy, to the truth (as best as it can be known at the time), and to keep yourself and your children safe and free of harm are very basic human rights.

What are my legal rights to "Informed Consent" and "Informed Refusal"?

Whenever a medical procedure, drug, test or other treatment is offered to you, you have the legal right to "informed consent". This means that your doctor, midwife or nurse is responsible for explaining:

◊ Why this type of care is being offered

◊ What it would involve

◊ The risks and benefits that are associated with this type of care

◊ Alternatives to this care, and their respective risks and benefits, including doing nothing (that is, simply waiting longer).

You have a right to clear and full explanations about your care. You are entitled to get answers to any and all questions that you may have about your care. You are also within your rights to request and receive a copy of your medical records and to get a second opinion.

Then, by law, you have the right to decide whether to accept the care that is offered. If you disagree with your caregiver and decide not to accept care that is offered to you, this is called "informed refusal". And, even if you have made your decision and signed a form agreeing to a particular type of care, you have the right to change your mind.

It can be challenging to carry out the informed consent process in the context of busy health care routines. Yet, you and your caregiver can set aside the time to discuss these issues in advance whenever possible and again when it is time to make a decision. You don't want to be learning about procedures and options for the first time when you're in labour and facing important decisions.

What are some tips for exploring these issues with my doctor or midwife?

Make a list of your questions before each visit, and take notes on the answers. You may wish to bring your partner or someone else close to you along to listen to what is said. Don't be shy; nothing is off-limits. While talking with your caregiver, don't hesitate to say:

◊ I don't understand.

◊ Please explain this to me.

◊ What could happen to me or my baby if I do that? Or if I don't?

◊ What are my other options?

◊ Where can I get more information?

◊ I have some information I'd like to share with you.

◊ I'm uncomfortable with what you are recommending.

◊ I'm not ready to make a decision yet.

◊ I'm thinking about getting a second opinion.

And remember, any question that you have is a question worth asking. It's important to let your caregiver know when you don't understand. Ask again, until you do.

What happens if my caregiver and I disagree?

Your caregiver has rights, too. He or she has the right to agree or disagree to provide care that you may request. For example, if you request a caesarean and have no medical need for this procedure, your caregiver has the right to refuse to do the surgery.

These issues speak to how important it is to have a good relationship with your caregiver that includes open communication, mutual respect, and shared points of view. Making a careful choice of a doctor or midwife who respects your needs, values and goals can help avoid conflict down the road.

© 2004 Maternity Center Association

Use your BRAIN to help you make informed choices

B — what are the **Benefits** of this (test, intervention, etc.)?

R — what are the **Risks** associated with this course of action?

A — what are my **Alternatives**?

I — what is my **Intuition** telling me?

N — what if we do **Nothing** or just wait a while?

How to Choose Your Caregiver

Many Western doctors hold the belief that we can improve everything, even natural childbirth in a healthy woman. This philosophy is the philosophy of people who think it deplorable that they were not consulted at the creation of Eve, because they would have done a better job. (Klooster-man, 1994)

We spend more time finding a good travel agent than we do, as mothers-to-be, finding the right caregiver to guide us through pregnancy and birth. Birth planning can determine if your current doctor/ midwife is the best match for you. But how can you find this out? If you are a private patient then it's easy – you just ask a few creatively worded questions. If you don't like the response you get, then you interview another doctor until you find one who is on the same page as you are. If you are a semi-private patient, your choices aren't as good. You'll meet a team of doctors and you have no idea who will show up on the big day, but you can still ask the questions. For public patients the options aren't much better because again you won't know who will be caring for you during your labour.

Team Edward or Team Jacob (Obstetrician-Led Care Versus Midwife-Led Care)

Depending on what's most important to you, both "teams" have a lot to offer – Consultant-led care just like Team Edward could be described as charming, polite and extremely protective, but on the downside just like Edward obstetricians tend to over-analyze situations and often overreact (seen in our growing rate of caesarean births). Bella describes Jacob as a "happy person" who extends this happiness to the people around him. Midwives trust birth and see birth as a life changing positive event in a woman's life rather than an accident waiting to happen. Women are most empowered and have the best experiences when both teams work collaboratively for the benefit of mum and baby (aka team Renesmee!)

Not all expectant mums will have access to the options below, and some options are available but not routinely offered at the GPs – so ask lots of questions!

◊ Hospital Birth Centre (Midwife-led unit): Drogheda and Cavan

◊ Hospital: Obstetrician

◊ Hospital: Community Midwives (for public mums only)

◊ Homebirth service (Community Midwives or self-employed community Midwives.

Obstetricians are trained in abnormal and complicated births. According to the World Health Organisation:

> Generally obstetricians have to devote their attention to high-risk women and the treatment of serious complications. They are normally responsible for obstetric surgery. By training and by professional attitude they may be inclined and indeed, are often required by the situation, to intervene more frequently than the midwife. In many countries, especially in the developing world, the number of obstetricians is limited and they are unequally distributed, with the majority practising in big cities. Their responsibilities for the management of major complications are unlikely to leave them much time to assist and support the woman and her family for the duration of normal labour and delivery. Obstetricians in many countries have concluded that care during normal childbirth should be similar to the care in complicated deliveries. This concept has several disadvantages: it has the potential to turn a normal physiological event into a medical procedure; it interferes with the freedom of women to experience the birth of their children in their own way, in the place of their own choice; it leads to unnecessary interventions; and, because of the need for economies of scale, its application requires a concentration of large numbers of labouring women in technically well-equipped hospitals with the concomitant costs. Staff in referral facilities can become dysfunctional if their capacity to care for very sick women who need all their attention and expertise is swamped by the sheer number of normal births which present themselves. In their turn, such normal births are

frequently managed with "standardised protocols" which only find their justification in the care of women with childbirth complications.

Midwives are trained in normal birth (about 80 per cent of all births). In an ideal world, you would never see a consultant (obstetrician) unless you had a problem in your pregnancy. All of your prenatal care would be undertaken by midwives. Seeing an obstetrician for a normal pregnancy is like taking a two-year-old to a specialist paediatrician any time he gets a cold.

All current research supports midwife-led care for low-risk pregnancies – the vast majority of pregnancies in Ireland. Unfortunately, maternity care is mostly obstetrician-led in Ireland. Fear forms a huge part of what is driving the current model of managed obstetric care. If we were not so terrified of our bodies and pregnancy from childhood – a terror bred through YouTube and One Born Every Minute – then it would make absolute sense for women to automatically choose a midwife when they become pregnant.

Similarly, there are essentially two very different ways of caring for a pregnant woman: **active management** (obstetrician-led) and **expectant management** (midwife-led). Many obstetricians and some hospital midwives see birth as a medical emergency, one that needs to be monitored continuously. In some hospitals in Ireland, this is tied to the notion that the success of your birth is purely dependent on whether you have efficient or inefficient **contractions**. Active management takes away the personal care that pregnant women need and reduces them to the numbers of contractions plotted on a chart. This is what's also known as the "production line" model of care.

According to the active management philosophy a woman's labour is only considered "normal" if she gives birth within the hospital's time limits — usually twelve hours. If you do not dilate according to the active management guidelines, you can expect to be encouraged to have your labour speeded up with artificial hormones. Which is fine if you've got someplace you need to be . . .

However, most women don't like to be rushed when we're doing something important, such as giving birth.

Expectant management care is generally practised by most community and independent midwives and a few consultants who see pregnancy and birth as a significant but normal part of a woman's life and have more of a "wait and see" attitude. A consultant or midwife with an expectant management approach will encourage you to be actively involved in your own care and to be fully engaged in all decision-making, will encourage birth plans and will expect you to ask questions. Caregivers with this philosophy will not routinely schedule **inductions** or break your waters. Expectant management means your labour is viewed as natural, unless there are medical signs that suggest otherwise, and that your body knows what to do. Your care provider follows your lead with no, or very little, intervention. On the other hand, an active management caregiver takes the active role and manages your labour through intervention.

Of course, it is not simply a matter of asking your consultant or midwife if they practise active management or expectant management. Some caregivers (and hospitals) may have very medicalised (active management) policies on certain issues, such as determining when they feel an episiotomy is necessary, while they may have a more expectant management philosophy on, say, whether or not to speed up or augment labour.

So, there are many points in between the "extremes" of active and expectant management. Only you can decide at what point you would feel most comfortable, and try to find a caregiver who is sympathetic to your needs. Read up (in this book and elsewhere) and become informed about inductions, caesareans, episiotomies, etc., and ask your caregiver relevant questions about their policies. If you are not happy that they are meeting your expectations, it is possible to change to a different caregiver. Of course, this is not easy to do when you're a public patient, which is why having a birth plan (see pages 54–58) is so important — on the big day, you won't know who will be there to help you birth your baby. If you're a private patient and seeing a consultant that it isn't working out, don't try to get your consultant to change

– change consultant! Talk to women who have had the kinds of birth you want and find out who their consultant was.

Choosing a Hospital

Established in the US in 1996, the Coalition for the Improvement of Maternity Services (CIMS) is a collaborative effort of numerous individuals and more than 50 organisations representing over 90,000 members. Their mission is to promote a "wellness model" of maternity care that will improve birth outcomes and substantially reduce costs.

A group of experts in birthing care came up with a list of ten things to look for and ask about. Medical research supports all of these things. These are also the best ways to be mother-friendly. Here's what you should expect, and ask for, in your birth experience. Be sure to find out how the people you talk with handle these ten issues about caring for you and your baby.

Ten Questions to Ask Your Hospital

1. Who can be with me during labour and birth?

Mother-friendly, midwife-led units, hospitals and home birth services will let a birthing mother decide whom she wants to have with her during the birth. This includes fathers, partners, children, other family members or friends (and should not be restricted to just one birth partner).

They will also let a birthing mother have with her a person who has special training in helping women cope with labour and birth. This person is called a doula or labour support person. She never leaves the birthing mother alone. She encourages her, comforts her and helps her understand what's happening to her.

They will have midwives as part of their staff so that a birthing mother can have a midwife with her if she wants to. The WHO is supportive of women having a choice in their birth supporters.

2. What happens during a normal labour and birth in your setting?

If they give mother-friendly care, they will tell you how they handle every part of the birthing process. For example, how often do they

---

give the mother a drug to speed up the birth? Or do they let labour and birth usually happen on its own timing?

They will also tell you how often they do certain procedures. For example, they will have a record of the percentage of C-sections they do every year. If the number is too high, you'll want to consider having your baby in another place or with another doctor or midwife.

Here are some numbers CIMS recommend you ask about:

◊ They should not try to start labour for more than one in ten women (10%) (37% of first-time mothers attending the Coombe will be offered induction of labour).

◊ They should not do an episiotomy on more than one in ten women (nearly half of all first-time mothers attending NMH will have an episiotomy).

◊ They should not do C-sections on more than one in ten women (10%) if it's a public hospital. According to the WHO, the rate should be no higher than 15% in hospitals caring for many high-risk mothers and babies. (Sadly Ireland is now approaching one in three women having surgical births, and close to one to two in some units.)

◊ Mothers who have had a C-section can often have future babies vaginally (VBAC). Look for a birthplace where at least 70% of women who opt for VBAC will have one.

3. How do you allow for differences in culture and beliefs?

Mother-friendly birth centres, hospitals, and home birth services are sensitive to the mother's culture. They know that mothers and families have differing beliefs, values and customs.

For example, you may have a custom that only women may be with you during labour and birth. Or perhaps your beliefs include a religious ritual to be performed after birth. There are many other examples that may be very important to you. If the place and the people are mother-friendly, they will support you in doing what you want to do. Before labour starts, tell your doctor or midwife special things you want.

4. Can I walk and move around during labour? What position do you suggest for birth?

In mother-friendly settings, you can walk around and move about as you choose during labour. You can choose the positions that are most comfortable and work best for you during labour and birth. (There may be a medical reason for you to be in a certain position.) Mother-friendly settings almost never put a woman flat on her back for birth. Jamie Oliver would call this an "organic" or "free range" birth.

5. How do you make sure everything goes smoothly when my nurse, doctor, midwife or agency need to work with each other? Can my midwife come with me if I have to be moved to another place during labour?

Mother-friendly places and people will have a specific plan for keeping in touch with the other people who are caring for you. They will talk to others who give you birth care. They will help you find people or agencies in your community to help you. For example, they may put you in touch with someone who can help you with breastfeeding.

6. What things do you normally do to a woman in labour?

Experts say some methods of care during labour and birth are better and healthier for mothers and babies. Medical research shows us which methods of care are better and healthier. Mother-friendly settings only use methods that have been proven to be best by scientific evidence.

Here is a list of things we recommend you ask about. They do not help and may hurt healthy mothers and babies. They are not proven to be best for the mother or baby and are not mother-friendly:

◊ They should not keep track of the baby's heart rate all the time with a machine (called an electronic foetal monitor). Instead it is best to have your nurse or midwife listen to the baby's heart from time to time.

◊ They should not routinely break your bag of waters early in labour.

◊ They should not use an IV (a needle put into your vein to give you fluids).

◊ They should not tell you that you can't eat or drink during labour.

A birth centre, hospital or home birth service that does these things for most of the mothers is not mother-friendly. Remember, these should not be used without a special medical reason.

7. How do you help mothers stay as comfortable as they can be? Besides drugs, how do you help mothers relieve the pain of labour?

The people who care for you should know how to help you cope with labour. They should know about ways of dealing with your pain that don't use drugs – this is true midwifery care. They should suggest such things as changing your position, relaxing in a warm bath, having a massage and using music. These are called comfort measures.

Comfort measures help you handle your labour more easily and help you feel more in control. The people who care for you will not try to persuade you to use a drug for pain unless you need it to take care of a special medical problem. All drugs affect the baby.

8. What if my baby is born early or has special problems?

Mother-friendly places and people will encourage mothers and families to touch, hold, breastfeed and care for their babies as much as they can. They will encourage this even if your baby is born early or has a medical problem at birth. (However, there may be a special medical reason you shouldn't hold and care for your baby.)

9. Do you circumcise baby boys?

Medical research does not show a need to circumcise baby boys. It is painful and risky. Mother-friendly birth places discourage circumcision unless it is for religious reasons. Fortunately this is not an issue in Ireland yet.

10. How do you help mothers who want to breastfeed?

The World Health Organisation made this list of ways birth services support breastfeeding:

◊ They tell all pregnant mothers why and how to breastfeed.

◊ They help you start breastfeeding within one hour after your baby is born.

◊ They show you how to breastfeed. And they show you how to keep your milk coming in even if you have to be away from your baby for work or other reasons.

◊ Newborns should have only breastmilk. (However, there may be a medical reason they cannot have it right away.)

◊ They encourage you and the baby to stay together all day and all night. This is called "rooming-in".

◊ They encourage you to feed your baby whenever he or she wants to nurse, rather than at certain times.

◊ They should not give pacifiers ("dummies" or "soothers") to breastfed babies.

◊ They encourage you to join a group of mothers who breastfeed. They tell you how to contact a group near you.

◊ They have a written policy on breastfeeding. All the employees know about and use the ideas in the policy.

◊ They teach employees the skills they need to carry out these steps.

© Coalition for the Improvement of Maternity Services (CIMS).
www.motherfriendly.org

Grainne's First Birth Experience

*T*he birth of my first baby took place at the beginning of last year in an Irish hospital. Following a routine visit, on a Wednesday, to my consultant (a stand-in, as mine was on holidays) from the scan she said she could see a decrease in the amount of fluid and was sending me in to be induced. She asked if I noticed a reduction in movements. I said yes but that I felt it was due to the baby growing, and that I still had movement.

However, she said that, based on this information and on her findings from the scan, I should be induced that night. Not knowing any different at that time, I agreed.

That night the consultant was too busy and I was told it would take place in the morning. All day Thursday I was monitored and the baby traced. Again, I think the delay was because they were too busy. I was even allowed into town to go shopping and told to come back to the hospital later that evening!

I was finally induced on Friday afternoon. It was never explained to me what this entailed, the effects on me or my baby or what I should expect. The first attempt was not happening quickly enough for their liking so I was given another half dose a while later. Following this, about 5.00 pm, the contractions came hard and fast. I requested the epidural as I was terrified. I was told I could go for it shortly. I had read that to be mobile helps, so I walked up and down corridors but I was in agony. I was then told by a midwife that a more urgent case had taken priority and I must wait a little longer for the epidural. I continued walking around for another few hours until I couldn't go on anymore and again asked about the epi. I was again told, "Sorry, but someone else has turned up and needed the delivery room so it'll be another while before we've a room free".

I continued alone and I was dilating ever so slowly but the pain was severe (as I found out later, induction makes the pain much more intense). Seven hours after I first asked about the epi, I called a midwife to find out what the situation was. She said she'd find out and a third time returned to tell me, "Sorry, but we're really busy tonight and someone else needed the delivery room again". She then said she could give me an injection of pethidine for the pain. I was in agony and agreed and so it was administered. Again, what this meant was not explained, nor were the effects mentioned. I only later found out about the risks to the unborn baby.

At 7.00 am the following morning I was eventually brought to the delivery section, but not to a suite, just to where I could use gas and air. I remained there for another few hours until a room came free. On examination by a registrar there, I overheard him say to a colleague, "She never had decreased waters." He left the room and I didn't see him again to pursue this, though I wasn't in the frame of mind to pursue it anyway. But of course if this was true I presume I would never have needed to be induced!

I was eventually brought into the delivery suite. Not long after I felt the need to push, and asked the midwife what to do. I was told to just push when I had a contraction so I remember trying to fight against pushes and it felt awful. She would also disappear out of the room for short periods, leaving just me and my husband. I had to get him to call the midwife when I thought I should push, as I wanted to make sure I was doing it properly. It was chaotic.

My recollection of the rest is still traumatic for me. After an endless time of pushing, where I felt my heart was going to explode (my husband later told me my face was as purple as could be; he thought I would burst), I told the midwife I didn't feel I could go on. I was so tired, had no energy left, was in horrendous pain and was starting to feel like a failure. The midwife told me she'd get the consultant.

So a male consultant appeared, examined me and then told me he'd be back to give me some help! When he returned he was armed with instruments and when he opened them out I nearly had a stroke. He then performed an episiotomy, without explanation or my consent, and proceeded to insert a vacuum, again without explanation/consent.

He asked me to tell him when I had a contraction. When I said one was coming the midwife shook her head as if to indicate I was wrong; the consultant asked the midwife "does she?" How demeaning! I definitely felt at this point as though I didn't have a clue, as I was even being told when I was or wasn't having a contraction, like I didn't know my own body! I insisted I had a contraction coming and the midwife said, "Well, I suppose she'd feel them first."

Eventually it ended and my beautiful baby girl was put on my chest for a moment. Although I say that now, at the time I was in such shock from this horrendous experience that I didn't even take it in. I was wheeled back to my room carrying my baby; I barely remember the journey I was so traumatised.

I now well up even recalling all of this. I feel that what should have been the most exciting and memorable time of my life was robbed from me by this despicable hospital experience.

I am now both saddened by it but also very angry. A short time ago I expressed my dissatisfaction in a letter to the hospital administrator. The response was that an investigation would take place; and the outcome of that was an apology, but not from anyone in particular. So I don't actually know who is sorry, but I know it's worded that way so no one is held accountable for legal reasons. Also, everything I described here was justified in his responding letter. So, with no real remorse from them I must just let it lie but am still very bitter and very afraid of ever becoming pregnant again. I obviously love my baby immensely and am delighted she is here.

<><><><><><><><><><><><><><><><><><><><><><><><><><><><><><><><><>

<><><><><><><><><><><><><><><><><><><><><><><><><><><><><><><><><>

Louise's Birth Story

My name is Louise and I would like to tell my "birth story". I am 29 and was due my second baby in March 2005. It was our older son's seventh birthday that day and he was really looking forward to his big birthday present. His birthday came and there was no sign of this little one coming. As I had my antenatal check-up that day my doctor asked me should he stretch the membranes a little. I was delighted as this had worked wonders on James and had started labour that time. And it worked again, albeit a little slower this time. I had very light contractions all night and couldn't sleep in anticipation of what would happen. I finally got up at 7.00 am and was disappointed as my contractions were still only very light and came only every 15 minutes. There was no way I was going to wait another day – this baby was coming out today and that was that!

So myself, my partner Conor and James all went for a long walk, then I took a bath and then went for another walk. At around 4.00 pm we dropped Max off at his granny's house and made our way to the hospital. There I walked some more. At 7.30 pm – after about six hours of walking – I was admitted. Conor went home for a while and I walked some more!

49

Finally at 11.30 pm, my waters broke. However, my contractions, although quite strong, were still very short, which meant my cervix was only dilating quite slowly. I went back up to the delivery room and was told .. . yes, to walk some more. Conor was massaging my back as I walked the corridors of the hospital, I can still see them in front of me!

By 1.00 am I had had enough. I was exhausted so I asked the nurse for the epidural. As I was 3 cm dilated at this stage the nurse agreed. However, while we waited for the anaesthetist, the baby's heart rate started to increase. This worried the doctor increasingly and we were told they would have to take blood from the baby's head. At this stage I was on gas and air but the contractions were about 45 seconds long and came every minute and a half. Conor had to leave the room and I can only imagine how worried he must have been for the next 15 minutes. They were the longest 15 minutes of my life! I knew deep down that there would be no time for the epidural, the contractions were too painful and too long and I already felt like pushing towards the end.

When the results came back from the lab the doctor was happy enough to give me the epidural, but after examining me he found I was 8 cm dilated so there was no time. I cried! I could not imagine going through this pain for the next hour. I needn't have worried: the second stage of my labour lasted only three minutes and after pushing three times, our beautiful baby girl was born at 3.18 am.

The cord was wrapped around her neck quite tightly and that was the reason she had been so distressed. She had also pooped in the womb just prior to birth, which again was an indication of how distressed she had been. She was put on my lap and I could not believe how similar she looked to her older brother — they were identical! I was in a daze, but looking at her I knew there was something wrong. Instead of breathing she was grunting and she was a bluish colour. I immediately panicked and kept saying: "She's not breathing, she's not breathing!" They examined her and gave her oxygen, but it took minutes until she stopped grunting. They then told us she would have to go to the ICU for a little while. Their information was very sketchy but they reassured us it was because she had been born too quickly and was nothing to worry about.

It is difficult to describe the feeling in that delivery room. The room was so empty and we had so many questions. Was she OK? Why did they rush her off? Was there something they were not telling us? Did she have brain damage? I think that was the biggie. Neither of us wanted to ask that question. We wouldn't have been ready for the answer. In what seemed like an eternity I got showered and dressed in my pyjamas and then we sat there waiting to be taken to ICU.

We finally went to see her at around 6.00 am. She was in an incubator with tubes everywhere and her eyes were wide open. She was looking at me, sucking on her fingers. I kept thinking, she's only so small, she can't understand why I'm not with her. I will never forget this incredible feeling of helplessness and this urge to just hold her. The doctors told us she had a pneumothorax, a collapsed lung and therefore she needed oxygen. The oxygen would help to reduce the air bubble which had escaped her lung into the chest. It was apparently very small so it wasn't too serious. It would take a day or two to clear. As there had been meconium in the womb they also wanted to give her antibiotics to avoid a possible infection.

There it was. It didn't sound all that serious but part of us was convinced they were trying to protect us and weren't telling us everything. There was nothing we could do. I had to leave my beautiful new baby "on her own" and go downstairs to my bed. I had such mixed feelings; I didn't know if she was going to be OK … Could she die? Was there permanent damage? …

She was on oxygen for two days and I was not allowed to take her into my arms for those two days. I couldn't even take her out to feed her. I had to express milk and they had to feed her through a tube into her nose. It was very hard to sit in the ward looking at the other new mums with their new babies and mine wasn't there. I cannot describe the joy I felt when I could finally take her down to the ward with me on the third day of her life. Finally she was there beside me and she was OK.

Isabel is now nearly six months old and she is the happiest baby ever! She has never been sick and the doctors have reassured us that there will be no lasting effects on her health. Although it was definitely not the labour of my dreams, she makes up for that a hundred times over!

Choosing Your Birth Partner

Your bag is packed. You've finally figured out the car seat and your partner has just finished assembling the cot with Krypton Factor-like precision. Your guess date is fast approaching. It's time to think about who can best support you during the exciting – and sometimes scary – hours of labour. Just as you carefully selected your consultant or midwife, your choice of birth partner is an important decision.

I'm sure you are aware of the old Hollywood cliché of the anxious expectant father pacing the corridors of the hospital, waiting for good news; his first glimpse of his new baby only coming when some smiling nurse holds the infant up to him from a glassed-in nursery. This was followed by the celebratory cigar. Thankfully, those days are long gone (if they ever really existed) and hospitals welcome birth partners, whether they are husbands, mothers, sisters, friends or even a doula (professional labour supporter). If you're having a doula you'll need to get permission from the head of obstetrics.

Mothers, sisters or friends who have already had babies often make good birth partners, if you are close to them. They will know most of what you are going through. Again, though, it is important that they are singing from the same hymn sheet as you – in other words, that they know and respect your choices. If your mother feels that her three caesareans were the best thing that ever happened to her, she may not be the best support if you are determined to achieve a vaginal delivery.

For the majority of women nowadays, however, their birth partner is usually their life partner. Today's fathers are, for the most part, very willing participants in their children's births — at least to the extent they can be! They may be the person most in tune with your needs, and they may be able to read signals from you that others cannot. Talk through your needs and expectations with your husband and partner, and ensure that they are happy with the role they will play.

From my own experience, dads are much more relaxed when they know that their partner is getting the special attention of a doula, especially if things get a bit messy. At a recent birth I supported, at one point dad was sitting in the corner with the blood pressure cuff on him, trying to take his own blood pressure! Hospitals with all their high-tech machines are like Toyland to many nervous dads. Once the pressure is off they can really relax and participate in a way that is most comfortable for them. Research shows that dads interact with mums more and touch them more when doulas are present. Doulas help fathers deal with the not-so-pleasant aspects of labour such as blood, pain and sheer unpredictability. Recent evidence has shown that the presence of a doula is associated with fewer medical interventions and shorter births, and that both mothers and babies have a more positive experience.

Post-natal doulas can also be a great help in the early days of parenthood. They can help with breastfeeding, newborn care and help new parents get some well-needed rest. This is especially crucial if the new parents have no family living nearby.

Here's what a good birth partner can do for you:

◊ Know your needs and be able to pass them on to the midwife or consultant

◊ Be informed of everything that might happen during the labour and delivery

◊ Be able to help you to relax

◊ Reassure you if things seem to be going differently to how you thought they would

◊ Help you to make important decisions at the right time, or to stick to your guns if it is in your best interest and that of your baby.

The Fear Factor

In a world where most first-time mothers' beliefs about birth are formed though horror stories from their mothers, sisters and friends, and endless reruns of reality birth shows, it's no wonder most mothers are terrified of birth and more are choosing to have caesareans. Fear slows labour. So how can you get past it?

Get informed. Read books that focus on birth being a positive experience. *Ina May Guide to Childbirth* is a great start and will really boost your confidence that birth is something that we women do very well. Just as you are more selective about what you put into your body during pregnancy, start being more selective about what you put into your mind. In a top 10 list of things to avoid when pregnant, I would put YouTube in the top 3. If you can't pull yourself away from YouTube search for "hypnobirth" or "GentleBirth" for a much quieter, calmer portrayal of birth. When Aunty Betty insists on telling you about her 54 hour labour ask her to wait until after you've had your baby. Talk to mothers who have had the kind of birth you'd like to have. Think about what you want to happen on the day rather than what you don't want. Take a class that gives you the tools to prepare for the best experience possible rather than to be the best patient possible.

Your Birth Preferences

Birth Plans and Fine Dining – A La Carte or Drive Thru?

If you've attended hospital antenatal classes you will have had the set menu, or what I call the drive thru menu, explained to you. What you probably don't know is that your hospital has another wonderful a la carte menu available too, but it's not advertised or promoted as much due to staff and bed shortages. But why should staffing problems affect your labour experience? You'd stop going to your favourite restaurant if they suddenly changed the menu and took all of your favourites off because the drive thru menu was quicker and more cost effective for the owner.

So What's on the Drive Thru Menu?

◊ Frequent vaginal exams to make sure you haven't deviated from the set timetable (dilating at 1 cm per hour)

◊ Your waters are broken at 3 cm or sooner to speed up labour

◊ Drips to speed up your labour if you don't keep up with the hospital timetable

◊ Continuous monitoring (much harder to move about)

◊ Epidural due to the drip making your contractions extremely painful and stressful for your baby

◊ Caesarean or forceps/vacuum to pull your baby out when the epidural affects pushing

◊ Episiotomy/severe tear. If you choose the set menu you have 12 hours or less to give birth

◊ Similar to going out on Valentine's Day – reservations are high and your table has been booked for several diners (as has your delivery room in the busier hospitals). Speed is of the essence but it's hard to relax and enjoy your special night out with staff haunting your table hoping to clear it as soon as possible.

Giving Birth à la Carte

Just like any dining experience you decide what appeals to you and if you're not sure then having a helpful midwife recommend an option to you can be priceless – they may suggest options to you that you may never have considered before to make your experience a positive one.

Assuming all things are normal, à la carte means there's no hurry . . . no time limits . . . you can choose not to have the drip and labour in your own time. You can decide that breaking the waters so early isn't for you. Midwives in MLUs and Community Midwifery programs are experts in a la carte birth and are a great resource in helping you choose what's right for you and your baby – rather than the drive thru menu that everyone else gets.

That's why putting some thought into what you want in labour is so important especially if you don't have access to an MLU or Community Midwife program. Having the drive thru menu just because it's all you've been offered often results in more inter-vention than is necessary and not as positive an experience. Yes, you'll probably have your baby quicker (drive thrus are all about speed) but your experience is less likely to be as positive had you known the à la carte options were available. Of course if speed is your main focus then drive thru can be very appealing.

Having no idea of what you want and choosing to just go with the flow means you let the staff choose the menu for you – that's exactly what you want if there is an emergency . . . they are the experts . . . but as most women have normal labours à la carte is usually the safest and most satisfying birth for you and your baby (and interestingly costs the hospitals a lot less).

Start thinking about your choices and how you can make this experience as positive as possible. Once you're in the queue for drive thru it's very hard to get out of it . . . you just follow the car ahead of you and hope for the best.

Comparing birth to a fine dining experience may be a stretch for a lot of mums, but ask yourself – do you want a drive thru delivery where you get what you're given and speed is the focus or the à la carte birth where it's about quality, safety and a positive experience. (I know what Gordon Ramsay would say . . .)

Why Write Birth Preferences?

> "Prepare for a no fault birth . . . If you confidently partici-pate in all the decisions made during your labour and de-livery – even those that were not in your birth plan – you are likely to look upon your birth with no blame and no regrets." – William and Martha Sears, *The Birth Book*

Birth preferences are not contracts or guarantees of what will hap-pen at your birth but it is a great way of organising your thoughts about the big day ahead and figuring out what's important to you on this special day. Of course, we can't control everything that happens during labour but there is a lot we can control.

If this is your first baby it's comforting to know what's ahead of you so you can decide how you want to handle different sce-narios. No matter how good your relationship is with your doc-tor or midwife, you do not know the midwives at the hospital and they don't know you so some concise birth preferences can really help your midwife understand how to support you best – after all she's employed by you!

Even if you're planning a home birth and know exactly who will be present at the birth, it is worthwhile to think about your preferences.

Writing some birth priorities helps you to look at different situations that can arise so you have an understanding of what your options are long before labour – so there are very few surprises when you feel well informed. Once you've considered your options you realize that even if things change during labour you still have options (in other words – Plan B).

Some mums shy away from writing birth preferences, especially if they have the mistaken belief that it's going to guarantee that specific things will or won't happen during labour – we all know that babies don't read birth plans. There aren't any guarantees in labour so if someone is expecting that a birth plan is going to guarantee that something will or won't happen then you could really be setting yourself up for disappointment.

It's not the birth plan itself that can cause disappointment in labour but your expectations and motivation for creating it.

I sometimes hear from mums who say, "as soon as I got to the hospital the birth plan went out the window". If you've done your homework and understand the offerings at your hospital in managing your labour (drive thru or a la carte) then this is highly unlikely to happen as you and your partner are sharing the decision making with your midwife/doctor – rather than having someone make all the decisions for you. Your midwife and doctor go home at the end of their shifts – you have to live with your decisions forever.

Following is an example of a birth plan template used by many Irish couples.

Sample Birth Preferences

John and I are looking forward to having a positive birth experience at x. Below are our birth preferences. We appreciate your support during this special time.

During the Birth

I would like to keep VE's to a minimum (i.e. on admission) and only at my request after that (unless there is a concern for my baby).

I prefer to labour and birth in any position that I find comfortable. I will ask for pain relief if I need it.

I prefer not to have an admissions trace or continuous monitoring unless there is a concern for my baby.

As long as labour progresses normally and my baby is doing fine I prefer not to have my membranes released or have my labour speeded up.

I prefer not have an **episiotomy**

When I am fully dilated, and assuming our baby is doing well, I would like to wait until I feel the urge to push before beginning the pushing phase.

After the Birth

Assuming everything is normal I prefer to have a natural third stage or at a minimum to allow the cord to finish **pulsating** before it is clamped/cut. I understand that this has significant benefits for my baby.

I will be breastfeeding so I would prefer to have continuous skin to skin contact with my baby and postpone weighing/routine exams etc. until after the first feed.

My partner would like to cut the cord after it has finished pulsating.

Special Circumstances

Should intervention become necessary we would appreciate being fully informed of all risks, benefits and alternatives.

If a caesarean becomes necessary, my partner will remain with me at all times. Time permitting I wish to have an **epidural** for anaesthesia.

Thank you in advance.

Helping Yourself to Complementary Therapies

Many women in Ireland fully embrace homeopathy, reflexology and seem to be very well versed in other natural "remedies" that may help with pregnancy complaints. This chapter looks at a number of possible aids to pregnancy and birth, including:

◊ Massage

◊ Acupuncture/Acupressure

◊ Aromatherapy

◊ Herbs

◊ Bach Flower Remedies

◊ Homeopathy

◊ GentleBirth

◊ Active Birth and Yoga.

Antenatal Massage

Antenatal massage is growing in popularity in Ireland. There is never going to be a better time to enjoy a massage than when you're pregnant. It is sheer bliss and, from personal experience, quite addictive once you try it. Swollen ankles are a thing of the past; back aches just melt away; and your baby also gets the benefits of all those happy hormones (**endorphins**) your brain creates from being really pampered. Antenatal massage therapists use a special table or pad with hollowed out areas to accommodate your belly and, often, your breasts as well, so you can lie face-down. For many of us, being able to lie face-down is a distant memory until after the birth. Some don't have the special tables, so you will lie on your side with several soft pillows to support you. If you haven't had a massage before you can keep your undies on if it makes you more comfortable. A really good massage therapist will be very skilful at keeping you "draped" in all the right places throughout your massage, so you can just focus on relaxing.

Benefits of Pregnancy Massage

◊ Emotional support and nurturing touch

◊ Relaxation and decreased insomnia

◊ Stress relief on weight-bearing joints, such as ankles, lower back and pelvis

◊ Neck and back pain relief caused by muscle imbalance and weakness

◊ Assistance in maintaining proper posture

◊ Preparing the muscles used during childbirth

◊ Reduced swelling in hands and feet

◊ Lessened sciatic pain

◊ Fewer leg cramps

◊ Headache and sinus congestion relief.

© www.pregnancytoday.com. Reprinted with kind permission.

Acupuncture/Acupressure

Acupuncture during pregnancy can be helpful for relieving nausea, boosting your energy and may reduce the need for induction of labour. Stimulating specific acupressure points by your midwife or partner during labour can help mums manage the sensations while encouraging efficient surges of the uterus.

Aromatherapy in Pregnancy

In a study by Ethel Burns, Midwives found essential oils to be highly effective in reducing anxiety and the perception of pain during labour. The smell of an apple tart baking can transport you back to Saturday afternoons at your Nan's house and instantly give you a feeling of comfort and wellbeing. Aromatherapy is all about using smells (aromas) to bring about physiological and emotional changes. We don't really understand how aromatherapy works, but our sense of smell is one of our most powerful senses. You've probably noticed that your sense of smell has really heightened during pregnancy and it will be even more evident during labour. Not all oils are safe to use during pregnancy; read all instructions carefully, and talk to a professional aromatherapist.

Morning Sickness

To help prevent morning sickness, diffuse petitgrain and mandarin oils in an electric vaporiser overnight or sprinkle the oils on a tissue to place by your bedside as you sleep. For me the only thing that could keep away the nausea was the smell of lemons. I would carry a bag of chopped-up lemons with me everywhere. I'm sure I looked very strange standing in the supermarket with my face in a plastic zip-lock bag sniffing lemons . . . but, hey, whatever worked.

Tired and Emotional

If you're feeling exhausted or very emotional, choose balancing lavender, geranium or bergamot oil for your diffuser. Even if you don't have essential oils at home there's a huge selection of products now that come with added lavender. A nice warm lavender bath can make your day.

Massage

The benefits of massage have already been outlined; add in a safe, relaxing essential oil to the mix, and you're in heaven! During the first three months, Mary Tighe from BirthingMamas.com recommends using "plain sweet almond oil or another carrier", especially if you suffer from morning, noon and night sickness. Lavender is a universal scent for calming the senses and can be used for a nice soak in the bathtub in the evening, especially if you are suffering from insomnia. Aromatherapy is growing in popularity as a tool for birth to help mum stay relaxed (anything has to be better than the smell of antiseptic). If you are planning on using essential oils during your birth, let your caregiver know..

Safety

Again, it must be stressed that not all oils are safe to use during pregnancy; check all labels and talk to yhour aromatherapist. Here's BirthingMamas.com again: "For use on the skin or in the bath, dilute essential oils using a maximum of two drops of essential oil per 10 ml (two teaspoonfuls) of carrier oil. Do not use neat essential oils on the skin."

Herbal Use for Pregnancy and Birth

The use of herbs during pregnancy and birth goes back hundreds of years when the "wise women" of the villages would create preparations for mothers based on recipes passed down through time. These were the earliest forms of medicine. Herbs are perceived as "natural" but their potency should not be underestimated, especially during pregnancy. It's very important not to self-prescribe any kind of medicine for yourself while pregnant, whether it's natural or over-the-counter, unless it comes from a reliable source. (I would not consider the internet a reliable source.)

There has been very limited research into the side effects of traditional herbal remedies although this probably has more to do with the fact that drug companies would not be interested in sponsoring such research; but there are many experienced midwives who swear by them. Herbs affect different women in different ways, so it's very important to seek the expertise of a qualified herbalist who specialises in remedies for pregnant and/or breastfeeding mums.

At some point in your pregnancy, someone may well ask you if you have started your raspberry leaf tea yet. This is a herbal tea that is thought to tone the muscles of the uterus, but the research has been limited to a few small studies in Australia. Over the last year or two, RLT has become a staple for many women in Ireland, often taken with the mistaken belief that downing bucketfuls of this woeful-tasting "tea" will get labour underway. You're more likely to end up with some serious bathroom visits rather than the desired outcome. Please let your midwife and/or doctor know if you are taking any kind of herbs during your pregnancy and labour.

For more information about herbs and pregnancy, including herbs to use during birth, to improve lactation, and to help the newborn infant, see *Wise Woman Herbal for the Childbearing Year* by Susan Weed (Ash Tree Publishing).

Bach Flower Remedies

Another wonderful tool that is safe to use at any time during pregnancy and birth are the Bach flower remedies (or essences). The flower remedies were discovered by Dr Edward Bach in the 1920s and are a safe, natural way of dealing with the negative emotions that he believed were the cause of illness. The remedies harmonise your mental state and enable you to think more positively. Some of the most used remedies are:

◊ *Mimulus*: A useful remedy if you feel afraid of the birth or pain or fear of there being something wrong with the baby.

◊ *Elm*: This is a great remedy if you feel doubtful of your ability to cope and are feeling overwhelmed and stressed.

◊ *Mustard*: For unexplained depression. Great for the baby blues.

◊ *Olive* is a must for the fatigue that so often comes during the first and third trimester.

◊ *Rescue Remedy*: This is the ideal remedy for labour to help ease panic and shock! It is a very calming remedy. A drop of Rescue Remedy rubbed onto your baby can also help him adjust to the shock of life outside the womb. Rescue Remedy cream can also be used on sore nipples. Apply as often as necessary. Before a feed, simply wipe the excess residue from your nipples.

Bach flower remedies are preserved in brandy, but the recommended dosage is two drops in a glass of water, so don't expect to get a buzz from the Bach flowers. You'd probably ingest the same amount of alcohol walking by the Guinness Brewery! If you're concerned about taking any alcohol during your pregnancy then just keep this in mind. There hasn't been any research conducted on the safety or effectiveness of Bach flower remedies during pregnancy and birth.

Homeopathy

Homeopathy is very popular in Ireland. All over the country women are comparing prices of arnica at their antenatal appointments and debating the best places to get their "labour kit". According to the World Health Organisation, homeopathy is the second most widely used form of medicine in the world.

How Does It Work?

Your homeopath will recommend certain "remedies" for you to take (often in the form of tiny sugar pills) depending on the symptoms you have. The treatments are based on the idea that a remedy can help a problem if it produces symptoms similar to the ailment (this is known as the "Law of Similars"). As homeopathy is quite safe, you can use it for children, adults and animals. The remedies themselves are made from minute plant and mineral extracts. Keep any strongsmelling aromatherapy oils away from your homeopathic remediesor they will lose their potency. Of course, it is wise to let your caregiver know if you are taking any homeopathic remedies and also to let your homeopath know if you're on any medication.

Some Uses for Homeopathy during Birth

◊ Induction: Caulophyllum and Cimicifuga (please consult with your caregiver before attempting any kind of induction)

◊ Turning a breech baby: Pulsatilla is a favourite (for more on breech birth, see pages 128–137)

◊ Arnica should be in every mother's birth bag; it's great for preventing bruising and can help you heal faster.

There are thousands of homeopathic remedies available. Have a consultation with a qualified homeopath so you can get the remedy that will have the most beneficial effect for you. You should never self-prescribe.

GentleBirth

Hypnosis for birth is shown to reduce the need for medication and results in shorter more manageable births for a high percentage of first time mums – see pages 92–98.

Active Birth or Yoga Classes

The object of active birth classes is to help you use movement and gravity to labour in a natural and effective way. Active birth is when a mother nstinctively moves into positions that help her cope with labour,by using natural position changes and gravity to help the baby through the birth canal. It should not be confused with "active management", which is the term used for a third party (your doctor or midwife) who manages your labour. Gentle movement in labour can ease pain and also help labour progress. Active birth classes borrow heavily from yoga techniques, adapted for pregnancy.

Active Birth Classes: What's Involved

Classes typically begin with stretches to increase flexibility, and you may then practise movements for use in labour. For example, you might stand upright and sway your hips, or kneel on all fours and move your hips in larger or smaller circles to relieve imaginary contractions. You will pay attention to your breathing during all movements and stretches – nothing complicated; you simply focus on breathing out in a slow and controlled fashion. It is important to practise these movements and breathing techniques often and regularly. The best way to do this is to attend classes as often as possible; this is much more effective than simply attending one class or

---

workshop on breathing techniques and hoping you can remember them when you are in labour.

When you have practised these movements so often that they become second nature, you may well find yourself automatically using them in labour. Because the movements and breathing patterns are simple, and you have practised them often, they can be very effective tools to help you labour. Active birth teachers and antenatal yoga teachers practise in most areas of Ireland; classes are normally held weekly.

© www.homebirth.org. Adapted and reproduced with kind permission.

Boogie for Birth

The latest craze for expectant mums is the Boogie for Birth classes. For mums who prefer a little more "zip" than "zen" and enjoy some light fun exercise during their pregnancy. Classes are tailored to the mums attending, and don't require any dance experience. Mums learn birth dance moves inspired by belly dance, African dance, ballet and Latin dancing. Mums also learn valuable birth preparation skills and comfort measures for an active birth.

Gentle Exercises During Pregnancy

Although you don't want to start a new exercise regime while pregnant, pregnancy isn't an excuse to lie on the couch for nine months. Staying active and fit during pregnancy will help you feel better and can even help shorten your labour. When exercising during pregnancy, you should:

◊ Avoid exercises that require you to lie on your back, such as sit-ups, after your twentieth week.

◊ Avoid exercising in very hot weather.

◊ Drink lots of water.

◊ Wear a good sports bra that supports your breasts.

◊ Never exercise to the point of exhaustion.

◊ Do Kegel exercises (or pelvic floor exercises) religiously. The pelvic floor supports the bladder, uterus, and intestines. The added weight of the uterus during pregnancy can stretch out that floor, causing either the intestines or bladder to drop down. This is one of the reasons that so many elderly women suffer from incontinence. Prevention is the best medicine. Kegels involve contracting and releasing the PF muscles, similarly to stopping the flow of urination. Tighten and relax the muscle quickly several times a day.

◊ Call a doctor if you develop serious symptoms, such as pain, dizziness, vaginal bleeding or fluid leaking from the vagina.

Pelvic Rock

This exercise is good for lower back ache. To do the exercise, get on your hands and knees and slowly arch your back like an angry cat, tilting your pelvis. Hold it for a moment; then relax your back to a normal position. Sometimes just wiggling your hips in this position can feel wonderful.

Tailor Pose
Sit comfortably on the floor and bring the soles of your feet together pressing down lightly on your thighs so you feel a gentle stretch.

All Illustrations © Janelle Durham (www.janelledurham.com)

What's wrong with this picture?

Imagine trying to restrict an elephant to give birth on her back...

It would probably require drugs and might lead to surgery

The same thing that's wrong with this one!

Imagine trying to restrict a woman to give birth on her back...

It would probably require drugs and might lead to surgery

Labour: Is This It?

You've imagined this day for a long time and now you're wondering, "Is this it?" If you are a first-time mum, then you may have a few false alarms and be worried that you won't know if you are really in labour. This chapter describes some of the usual signs that things are starting to happen and labour is about to get under way. Sometimes things will happen at once, while for other mothers labour gets underway more gradually. But no matter how your labour begins, staying as relaxed as possible will help things progress much more quickly and less stressfully.

Don't be surprised if in the last few days of your pregnancy your energy comes back in bursts. You may have what some mothers refer to as the "nesting instinct". You may feel the need to get things organised and clean the house from top to bottom; this is very normal, so let your partner know you haven't totally lost the plot!

Labour: Recognising the Signs

In the first stage of labour, the cervix dilates from a closed position to 10 cm, when it is said to be fully dilated. In most Irish hospitals you are not "officially" in labour until you reach 3 cm. If you get to the hospital and are less than 3 cm, if everything else is as it should be, the best thing to do is to go home and relax; check this with your hospital. It can take up to 12 hours for the cervix to become fully dilated, although this is very individual; some mothers dilate more quickly than others.

Contractions

What are they?

Contractions are regular tightenings of the uterine muscles and occur throughout labour. During the first stage, these contractions help to dilate the cervix. In the second stage, they help to push the baby down the birth canal and in the third stage, the contractions also help deliver the placenta. When your contractions start, many first-time mothers mistakenly believe that they need to do 50 laps around the block to keep things moving and then find they are exhausted two hours into labour!

For labour to progress, it is important to reduce the adrenaline in your system; physical activity and stress increase adrenaline and reduce the "feel-good" hormones (endorphins). For more on this, see pages 84–86. In the early stages especially, try to conserve your energy and relax as much as possible. If you're a first-time mother, this is going to be hard because of all the excitement; that's why it's so important to practise some relaxation techniques long before you go into labour. For any birth partners reading this, it's up to you to help mum stay relaxed. Turn down the lights, run a warm bath for your partner or get the shower going – and above all, stay calm.

How do they feel?

Women experience contractions in a variety of different ways. Some say that they feel like very bad period pains in the stomach. Others describe the feeling as that of extreme constipation and wind. Sometimes, contractions appear to originate from the back and radiate towards the front. Contractions may also be accompanied by backache, nausea and/or diarrhoea. If you're having a homebirth, call your midwife and let her know what's going on.

What do I do?

Resist the temptation to text everyone, update your Facebook page or Tweet your progress – once the cat is out of the bag that labour has started all eyes are on you and you can do without the performance anxiety! If the sensations become more regular or start to increase in intensity call your midwife or hospital if you'd like some reassurance, especially if you are planning on staying home to labour as much as possible. If it's during the middle of the night try to rest as much as you can. If you have a relaxation CD put that on and keep your anxiety levels down. Consider having a bath or shower to relax you and keep you comfortable.

How do I time contractions?

When timing contractions, you need to be aware of two things:

how frequent and how strong the contractions are. Start the timer when you get the first contraction. The time when it ends is used to determine the duration of the contraction. When the second contraction starts, use the interval between the start time of this contraction and the start time of the previous contraction to determine the frequency of contractions. There's even an iPhone app available – Contraction Master!

Remember that many people wrongly time contractions as the interval between the end time of the first and the start time of the next contraction.

In a first pregnancy, the cervix is closed throughout. As labour begins (usually unnoticed) your cervix begins to efface (thin out) and dilate (open) when it is ripe and ready for your baby to be born.

A "Birth Show"

What is it?

A protective plug of mucous seals the cervix at the neck of the uterus throughout pregnancy. This plug begins to come away and passes down the vagina as a bloodstained discharge. This is called a "show".

When does it happen?

A show may occur several days before labour or it may even occur during the first stage of labour.

Your Membranes Release

Throughout pregnancy your baby floats in a sac containing amniotic fluid, or "bag of waters". When your baby is ready to be born, the membranes of this amniotic sac release causing the amniotic fluid to flow out of the vagina.

What will I feel?

You will either feel the fluid trickling or a sudden gush of fluid out through the vagina. Most commonly, there is a trickle if the baby has engaged by this time and its head has the same effect as a cork in a bottle.

When does it happen?

Your waters may release or "break" several hours before the onset of labour or this may occur during labour itself. For some women their waters will release and labour doesn't kick in for a while; this is normal. You don't have to worry about your baby; your body continues to produce amniotic fluid. Some babies are even born "in the caul" (the waters don't release until the moment the baby is being born). If your membranes release before 37 weeks, however, you should contact your caregiver immediately.

What to do?

If the fluid is clear, wear a sanitary towel if it makes you feel more comfortable. Call your midwife or the hospital. If the fluid is greenish, yellow or brown in colour, it may be a sign that the baby is in distress. This coloured fluid is actually due to the baby having passed meconium, its first stool, which would normally not happen until after birth. Call your midwife or hospital immediately.

Going to the Hospital

Staying home as long as you are comfortable is a great idea. Being in your own environment will help you deal with labour much better than being in the strange environment of the hospital with bright lights, noise and strangers. You'll feel much more relaxed at home, which is essential for helping your labour progress. If at any time you feel that something isn't quite right or have bleeding or your waters change colour, go to the hospital, or call your midwife if you're having a homebirth. Most hospitals recommend coming in once contractions are consistent and lasting at least 60 seconds every five to seven minutes. Your partner should bear in mind the distance from the hospital and traffic conditions, especially if you think you may need to leave for the hospital in the early morning or evening rush hour. It might not be a bad idea to do a "dry run" to the hospital some evening and see how long it takes you (partners: keep the car filled up!).

Premature Labour

What is it?

When labour starts before 37 weeks of pregnancy, it is termed as premature labour.

Why does it happen?

A history of premature birth, high temperature, or a multiple pregnancy all contribute to a premature labour. Unfortunately, premature labour is hard to predict.

How will I recognise the signs?

The signs of a premature labour are more or less similar to real full-term labour, as discussed above. It also depends on the prematurity of the labour; if you are close to 37 weeks, signs will be almost identical to a proper labour, whereas if you are many weeks behind, you may experience just a low back pain with or without contractions.

How is the baby affected in a premature labour?

Most babies born before 24 weeks won't survive. However, if born between 24 and 30 weeks, your baby will be very immature but will be able to survive in a special care unit. If your baby is born anytime after 34 weeks, he may be able to survive even without special care. If your caregiver is successful in stopping premature labour, you may be advised to either stay in hospital or at home on strict bedrest.

A premature baby's lungs are very immature and can cause major problems as the lungs don't know how to breathe. If there is a risk of your baby being born prematurely, steroids may be given to you which reach across to the baby through the placenta and help the baby's lungs to develop rapidly.

What happens if I go into premature labour?

◊ Attempts may be made to stop the contractions temporarily, either through the use of drugs for 48 hours or through antibiotics if you have an infection with a high temperature.

◊ You may be given an injection (such as pethidine) to calm you down.

◊ If you are dehydrated, a drip may be given to replenish your fluids.

◊ You will be advised to take steroids to speed up the development of your baby's lungs; this takes 24 hours to take effect.

◊ A premature labour is much quicker than a full-term labour, mainly because the baby is smaller.

© *Adapted and reproduced with the kind permission of*
www.mothersbliss.com

WHAT TO BRING TO THE HOSPITAL

A lot of mums live in the hope they'll go early. So the bags are packed and ready to go by the sixth month, if not sooner! Only five per cent of babies are born on their "guess date". It's probably a good idea to have your bags ready by 37 weeks, which is considered to be full term (anywhere between 37 and 42 weeks).

For Mum

◊ This book

◊ Birth plan (have a few copies)

◊ Light dressing gown

◊ Mobile phone and charger

◊ TENS machine

◊ Hand-held fan

◊ Lip balm

◊ Hair scrunchies or clips

◊ Antibacterial wipes (especially if you're sharing a bathroom with four other new mums)

◊ Flipflops (same reason as the wipes)

◊ Breast pads

◊ Slippers

◊ Two pairs of socks (you might not need them because hospitals are usually very warm)

◊ Old nightie (not essential as you'll be given a gown anyway, but it's nice to be in your own clothes)

◊ Three pairs of pyjamas, or a couple of tracksuits (you'll feel better being dressed)

◊ Toothbrush and toothpaste

◊ Shampoo and conditioner

◊ Deodorant

◊ Shower gel

◊ Two packs of sanitary towels (industrial strength with wings) or maternity pads

◊ Two towels

◊ Sponge or face cloth

◊ Big old granny knickers or disposables

◊ MP3 player

◊ Eye mask

◊ Going home outfit (something loose and comfy)

◊ Rescue remedy

◊ Arnica

◊ Lansinoh cream for breastfeeding

◊ A good nursing bra and a pair of pyjamas designed for breast-feeding

◊ Snacks (for labour for you and partner).

For Baby

◊ Car seat

◊ Six vests

◊ Six babygrows

◊ Five bibs

◊ Two soft towels

◊ One pack of newborn nappies

◊ Soother (not recommended if you are breastfeeding to avoid nipple confusion)

◊ Cotton wool

◊ Sudocreme

◊ Scratch mits and hat

◊ Outfit and blanket for going home (partner can bring this in on the day you leave).

Partner

◊ Fill up the car with petrol

◊ Change for parking

◊ Mobile phone (with credit)

◊ List of numbers

◊ Camera and film

◊ Sandwiches and snacks (fruit bars).

INDUCTION

There can be many varied reasons for your care provider wanting to induce your labour. In Ireland the rates vary from 10 per cent to a whopping 45 per cent! If you have shown signs of pre-eclampsia (high blood pressure and protein in your urine), your doctor may not want to wait for you to go into labour on your own if he or she feels there is danger in waiting. Other reasons for induction can include if your pregnancy goes over 40 weeks (most hospitals will be fine waiting 10–14 days past your guess date – see below) or if your waters break and you haven't gone into labour within a certain timeframe. There can be other reasons for a medical induction, such as health complications of the mother, but those are the most common.

When You Are Overdue

So 40 weeks have come and gone; you feel like you've been pregnant forever; no shows, no leaks and not a single contraction. Eviction is starting to look appealing.

Your estimated due date (EDD) is just that – an estimate – it is not an appointment, an expiration date or a best before date! It is based on a nineteenth-century formula called Naegele's Rule, which assumes that ovulation occurs on day 14 of a 28-day cycle for all women. We now know this to be incorrect. Your baby is considered to be full term anywhere from 37–42 weeks. Only 5 per cent of babies are born on their due date. Women generally assume they are overdue once they go past 40 weeks, but they are not actually overdue until reaching 42 weeks.

When you are already past your estimated due date (EDD), your care provider may suggest inducing your labour. Remember that only five per cent of babies are born on their due date. Some care providers suggest inductions based on the size of your baby. Ultrasounds are notoriously inaccurate. Think how difficult it is to estimate the weight of a baby you are physically holding – now try it with a black and white photo! Contrary to popular belief, the camera doesn't add 10 lbs – especially to ultrasound images!

Although it's tempting to know exactly when your baby will be born, inductions should never be done if the reason is that you are tired of being pregnant or want to have your baby on a specific date, or simply for the convenience of a doctor's holiday schedule. An induction comes with varied risks, depending on what type of stimulant is used to attempt to induce labour. Usually you can find out if you are a good candidate for induction by having your doctor give you a **Bishop Score**. This is a system that takes into account the position of the baby, the softness and readiness of your cervix, as well its position, to rate if an induction is more or less likely to work. It is recommended that an induction only take place if your Bishop Score is above 9.

Inductions are generally more painful than "normal" labour as your body doesn't have the ability to adjust to the natural start of labour. Your endorphins don't have a chance to catch up to labour that has been artificially started. If induction is being suggested because of low amniotic fluid levels at full term you can increase them by staying well hydrated. Water is a pregnant woman's best friend.

Induction Methods

In consultation with your care provider, you can use "natural induction methods" or medical induction methods. It is not recommended to try natural induction methods before reaching 40 weeks, and you should always discuss any method you want to try with your care provider before attempting it. In fact, "natural" is a bit of a misnomer. Any form of induction, whether it is "natural" or not, is an attempt to artificially kickstart labour. You will probably get lots of "advice" from your friends on the best way to do this, including sex, acupuncture, eating spicy food, walking, eating fresh pineapple . . . the list goes on. And it may seem like some of these methods work, but there's no proof that Auntie Orla wouldn't have gone into labour anyway, even if she hadn't cleaned out the local takeaway of their Madras "special"!

Here are how some common induction medications work, as well as their risks and possible side effects:

 ◊ **Prostaglandins**: These are synthetic (artificial) hormones which can be inserted into the vagina as a gel or removable tab in order to soften the cervix and make it ready for labour/induction. The risks include possible hyperstimulation of the uterus and possible foetal distress, which could lead to a c-section.

 ◊ **Oxytocin** (also known as syntocinon or pitocin or pit): This drug is given by IV in order to make the uterus start contracting. It is routinely used to speed up labour in some hospitals. Side effects of pitocin are: uterine hyperstimulation, foetal distress, low **Apgar scores** (suggesting oxygen deprivation) at birth, postpartum blood loss and neonatal jaundice. In first-time mothers, the use of pitocin increases the likelihood of having a c-section.

 ◊ **Stripping or sweeping your membranes**: Beginning at your 38-week appointment, your care provider may suggest a vaginal exam every week to gauge the progress of your cervix and to check to see if you are dilated at all. While this can give you hope (if you are slightly dilated) that you will go into labour soon, it is no real indication of when labour will start. Sometimes you will be 1–2 cm dilated for weeks before going into labour. Sometimes during these vaginal exams, your doctor may strip or sweep your membranes (with your consent of course). What this means is that he/she may (if you are more than a small fingertip dilated) sweep their finger around the inside of your cervix to separate your bag of waters from the entrance to your cervix. This is believed to release your body's natural prostaglandins in order to possibly start labour. While this may sound like a great idea if you are feeling ready to not be pregnant anymore, make sure to ask your doctor if they routinely do this procedure and ask them not to do it to you. Your risk of infection increases with any foreign object being inserted into your vagina. It is also possible to rupture your membranes accidentally, which comes with its own complications.

It is very important when selecting a caregiver that you are comfortable with his/her induction policies. If you are considering an induction it is important to understand the risks involved. Starting the induction process on a mother whose body is not ready to give birth can cause more problems than it solves. Midwives and doulas often describe a "cascade of intervention" when the natural flow of the birthing process is disrupted (see page 122). One intervention leads to another and often the end result is what you were originally trying to avoid – a caesarean.

Pain Management in Labour

Although the epidural is often described in degrees of bliss, there is no perfect drug. All drugs have the potential to affect you and your baby. It's ironic that we spend nine months swearing off drink, cigarettes, coffee and even hairdye and then we want the epidural waiting in the car park! When considering your options, think about how you currently deal with pain. When you have a headache, do you immediately reach for the paracetamol, or do you take a nice bath or have your partner rub your head?

In general, women think of labour pain as one continuous excruciating ordeal. This is reinforced by comments from friends such as, "You don't get a medal for not taking the drugs". However, labour pain is not like the pain you get when you break your leg. Breaking down the contractions makes it much more manageable. Let's say you're well into active labour and things are progressing perfectly. Even at the height of your contractions, chances are you'll be having a 90-second contraction every five minutes. That sounds like a lot, but let's break it down. The contraction is made up of three stages: the build-up, the peak and the release. In a 90-second contraction, the first 30 seconds are when you feel the contraction starting to build. Take a nice deep breath and you can focus all of your attention on the next 30 seconds – the "peak". After those 30 seconds are over, the contraction ebbs away and you can rest for another five minutes. So essentially you only have to deal with severe pain for 30 seconds, every five minutes. In one hour, that is 12 contractions multiplied by 30 second "peaks", which is only six minutes each hour that you really have to focus on. And the contractions usually only get that intense towards the end! Is that so awful?

Methods of Managing Pain

Epidural

Getting an **epidural** can in itself be an exercise in futility, depending on which hospital you're in. You'll be warned by everyone: don't get it too early . . . and don't get it too late! To "get" the epidural, you will need to sit or lie with your back rounded over (like the hunchback) for up to twenty minutes while an anaesthetist inserts a **catheter** into your back (see page 109). You will not be allowed to move during the insertion – not exactly easy when you're having a contraction so as soon as you feel one coming on tell the anaesthetist and he will stop until it's over. Your partner might do well to sit in front of you and hold your hand; watching an epidural procedure can make you queasy.

The epidural is not just a quick needle in the back. Once you've had the first intervention of an epidural there are others that follow suit: you have to have a drip to keep your blood pressure up; you have to be continuously monitored, and you will most likely be on your back for a considerable length of time. Ask the midwives to shift you on to your side every hour or so. It is ironic that throughout pregnancy mothers are advised not to sleep on their backs because it can restrict the blood flow to the baby – and yet that's how you end up sometimes for a long time when you have an epidural! Another common side effect from epidurals that is still "in the closet" so to speak is that once every muscle in your body has been anaesthetised you cannot control any excess gas that needs to exit – so prepare for some rippers! Don't worry, though, it's quite normal, even if it is quite mortifying when you aren't expecting it.

The epidural has been equally praised and damned by labouring women. For some, it is a positive experience, the pain relief allowing for a more relaxed birth experience. For others, however, the loss of control can be frustrating at best, and for some the epidural slows down and complicates what might otherwise be a straightforward labour. Some mothers lose the urge to push and have to have a vacuum or forceps delivery. Some mothers can develop a fever.

81

Babies are also affected by epidurals. Often the decision to accept an epidural is made without an awareness of these and other significant risks to both mother and baby. These risks are explained in more detail in the next chapter (page 110).

Narcotic Analgesics

While the epidural is a locally acting anaesthetic, narcotic pain-killers such as pethidine act to reduce the entire body's sense of pain.

Pethidine is the most common drug given in Irish hospitals. It works very much like morphine. It is usually given as an injection in the thigh or buttock, or sometimes as a drip, takes about twenty minutes to start working and lasts about two to three hours. Pethidine can make you sleepy and trippy. The problem with pethidine, apart from its side effects (see below) is that it seems to affect women in different ways. For some, the pain relief is minimal, or may only work early in labour, while others can be left feeling totally spaced out, distressed or feeling a complete lack of control. Remifentanil is becoming more popular for pain relief as it is fast acting with fewer of the side effects associated with Pethidine.

Specific risks of pethidine include:

◊ It can cause nausea

◊ You may need a drip

◊ It can slow labour causing a need for pitocin/syntocinon to speed it up again (which increases your risk of caesarean)

◊ You'll need continuous foetal monitoring, which decreases your mobility (probably not a bad thing if you're tripping on pethidine anyway)

◊ Like any drug, it might not work

◊ It affects the baby both before he's born and after through your breastmilk, so he may not show any interest in breastfeeding.

If your labour is progressing normally you probably won't have the option of pethidine if you are getting close to actually giving birth because the drug can affect the baby's breathing. Your body's natural endorphins are 200 times stronger than morphine, and come with no negative side effects – see below.

Taking the Edge Off: Entonox (Gas and Air)

Entonox, commonly known as "gas and air", is a mild painkiller consisting of oxygen and nitrous oxide, inhaled through a mask or mouthpiece. When you feel a contraction coming on, you take a nice deep breath and by the time the contraction peaks you should have some relief; it doesn't completely take the pain away but will take the edge off. If you find it makes you queasy or dizzy you can just stop using it. There has been little research done on the long-term effects of gas and air on mothers and babies.

TENS Machine (Transcutaneous Electrical Nerve Stimulation)

Transcutaneous means "through the skin". **TENS** machines (available for rent in Boots Chemists) deliver small electrical pulses to the body via electrodes placed on the skin. The sticky patches are placed on your back. It looks like those tummy-trimming devices that were popular a few years ago. Think of it like internet broadband – your spinal cord can only carry so much information to the brain and if its capacity is used up with electrical stimulation from the TENS machine, there's no room for the pain signals to get through. TENS doesn't work for everyone; some mothers find it very distracting, but at least it's self-administered and you can turn it up as you need it. If you don't like it, you can just take off the patches. There are no known side effects to using TENS, but you have to wonder if applying electrodes to your body affects the brain and that precise orchestration of hormone release that helps birth progress.

The Secret to an Easier Birth:
How Your Hormones Affect Birth

To make birth easier and labour shorter, it's critical to ensure the birth hormones are encouraged to do their job effectively. Four major hormonal systems are active during labour and birth. These involve oxytocin, the "hormone of love" (Michel Odent); endorphins, the "feel good" hormones; adrenaline, hormones of excitement and stress; and prolactin, the mothering hormone. These hormones are common to all mammals. For birth to proceed easily the primitive (instinctive) brain must take over from the front part of your brain (the thinking part). This occurs naturally and is helped by an atmosphere of quiet and privacy, with dim lighting and little conversation or distractions. Under these conditions, a mother will instinctively choose the movements, sounds, breathing, and positions that will birth her baby most easily. Creating this atmosphere in hospital isn't easy, but a CD player with calming music and an eye mask can be very helpful.

Endorphins and high levels of adrenaline cannot co-exist in labour. If there is an excess of adrenaline, then the body's own pain-killers (endorphins) are not present. Likewise if endorphin levels are increased, adrenaline levels lower, which makes for a much more comfortable labour.

Oxytocin

Oxytocin is the hormone that sends signals to your body to start contracting. It has also been shown to affect how we bond with others. Right as your baby is about to be born you have the highest levels of oxytocin in your body than at any other time in your life.

Endorphins

Your body's natural pain relievers are more powerful than morphine (and pethidine). Like oxytocin, endorphins are secreted from the pituitary gland, and high levels are present during sex, pregnancy, birth and breastfeeding. Beta-endorphin is also a stress hormone, released under conditions of duress and pain, when it acts as an analgesic.

Fight-or-Flight Hormones

The hormones adrenaline and noradrenaline are also known as the fight-or-flight hormones or, collectively, as catecholamines. They are secreted in response to stresses such as fright and anxiety, as well as excitement, when they activate the sympathetic nervous system for "fight or flight". We've all experienced this "fight or flight" phenomenon. Millions of years ago, it helped us survive attacks by wild animals. Obviously, for most of us that's no longer a threat, but it's a part of our primitive brain that remains with us. Your body has a physical response to a fright, whether it's real or imagined. How many of us have driven over the speed limit and then spotted a garda car behind us, lights flashing? Remember how your breathing increased . . . your heart raced . . . your hands became sweaty . . . and you probably felt physically sick for a few seconds . . . then the garda car overtook you, speeding off after someone else! While you were reading this your breathing rate probably went up too; the very thought of this scenario created a physical response. That's the effect of adrenaline on the body.

In the first stage of labour, high stress levels inhibit oxytocin production, thereby slowing labour. Adrenaline also acts to reduce blood flow to the uterus and placenta, and therefore to the baby, because the uterus is not a defensive organ. Reduced blood flow means muscles tire quickly. For animals giving birth in the wild, this response is important – the presence of danger would activate this sympathetic response and stop labour until the animal has moved to a safe place to birth or the threat has passed. Unfortunately, the subconscious mind does not differentiate between real and perceived fears for humans, so for most mothers the fight-or-flight response is redundant in labour. You're in a vulnerable position; you can't fight and you can't flee. So your body does the next best thing – it freezes. You may have heard the term "FTP", or failure to progress . . . In humans, high levels of adrenaline are associated with longer labour and adverse foetal heart rate patterns.

After an undisturbed labour, right as the baby is about to be born, these hormones act in a different way. There is a sudden increase in adrenaline levels, which activates the foetal ejection reflex, allowing the baby to be born in a few strong, uncontrollable contractions.

Ways to Optimise the Benefits of Your Birth Hormones

Because the slightest disturbance can affect the delicate balance of hormones during birth, the following are essential to help labour progress easily and quickly:

◊ Anything that helps you stay relaxed during your pregnancy is helpful (e.g. meditation, visualisation or yoga), particularly if you have been practising them over weeks or months.

◊ Create an atmosphere where you feel safe, unobserved and free to follow your own instincts.

◊ Reduce physical activity. Activity increases adrenaline in the body which leaves no room for those feel-good hormones. Don't fall into the trap of walking a marathon in labour unless you feel like walking. Being upright has the benefit of helping your baby into a good position, but follow your body's lead – nobody else's. If it feels good to walk, then walk.

◊ Reduce mental stimulation by keeping lighting low and keeping questions and distractions to a minimum (bring your CD player and eye mask). Relaxation is key.

© *Sarah Buckley, www.sarahjbuckley.com. Adapted and reproduced with kind permission from an article by Sarah Buckley MD*

OLD SCHOOL CHILDBIRTH

It's almost taboo to talk about having a natural birth in Ireland, it's like a secret society (it's like Fight Club . . . nobody talks about it). If you accidentally have a natural birth, that is, you gave birth so quickly you didn't have time for an epidural, you'll hear a collective groan of "OMG that's my worst nightmare – I hope you complained!" If you are actively considering a drug-free birth you'll soon be on the receiving end of comments about root canals without anaesthesia, medals and martyrs. I recently came across the term "old school childbirth" – it's much more hip and doesn't seem to raise hackles nearly as quickly. Old school conveys a positive attitude of an idea from years gone by that is still held in high esteem today. Of course not everyone "gets" why old school birth is so important to some mums, especially when there are so many options in how we give birth these days. Mountaineers can spend years preparing for a climb when they could just as easily take a helicopter to the summit, but for them climbing that mountain has huge meaning.

Claudia Panuthos explores the idea of natural birth in her book *Transformation through Birth*, written in 1984. Below is a quote that resonate with women preparing for an old school natural birth, also discussed on Molly Remer's "Talk Birth blog".

> "In some sense, childbirth is much like a marathon. Once given some general guidelines, marathon runners know how to breathe, to run, and to complete their race according to their own body signals. Similarly, women know how to breathe, to birth, and to complete the delivery according to their own body signals. Marathon runners who are true champions are free to stop the fast pace, and even quit the race without loss of integrity."

Panuthos then makes the point that birth is really more like a "Zen marathon" in that "the focus is to become centered and one with the body, to remain on purpose and directed toward a single goal and to act from the witness or higher mind within" and goes on to say, "Because we view marathon running as an expression of ultimate physical health, a similar attitude toward childbearing may greatly aid in the altering of present attitudes that respond to childbearing as an abnormal condition requiring medical treatment."

The marathon analogy really illustrates how the sensations of birth are not like the sensations of a broken bone or horrible illness. The sensations come and go. There is nothing "broken" with birth (well, usually)! The sensations of giving birth are more similar to the feeling of healthy muscles working hard and working for a long time, and doing something of which they are fully capable.

Some well meaning friends or family will say, "It's only one day in your life – in three months time you'll be pushing your baby in a pram, it doesn't matter how you gave birth once you have a healthy baby – what difference does it make?!" Would anyone say that to a marathon runner, or someone who has just won a Gold medal in the Olympics (analogy side note: feeling good that you won a Gold medal [gave birth in a triumphant and empowering way] does not invalidate or cause guilt in those who did not run the marathon, or had to quit early, or needed help finishing. There is no shame in not running, but there is also rightful pride and "glory" in finishing the "race" you set out on.)

Ways to be Active During Labour

The following illustrations are examples of what a mother will instinctively do during labour. Only move about if you feel you need to, not because someone suggests it. Sometimes when the baby is moving down through the pelvis he may put pressure on a certain muscle or nerve. You will automatically counter that pressure by changing position. So there's no need to memorise positions; you'll just do it!

Position Changes

The way in which your body is positioned during labour can make a huge difference in how manageable labour can be. It is not natural to lie down and stay still when you are uncomfortable. Think of the last time you stubbed your toe; instinctively you probably hopped around swearing like a trooper and rubbing it furiously. The same principles apply in birth. You will instinctively get into positions that feel best for you. Some positions improve your baby's ability to navigate through the pelvis; other positions make it harder for him. Some positions can help to reduce the pressure associated with a back labour (on all fours); other positions make it easier to relax your body and rest (side lying). Remember, if you are having a drug-free birth your body will tell you what to do; you just have to follow its lead. It is also important to understand that some medical interventions will limit your ability to change positions. If you have an epidural you will be confined to bed (on your back or on your side).

Birth balls are great to have before birth, just to sit on and rock; during birth to help the pelvis open up and take the pressure off the perineum; and after birth to bounce on with your baby and tone up your stomach muscles. During labour you can sit on the ball and have your partner massage your lower back.

All Illustrations © Janelle Durham (www.janelledurham.com)

Positions for Resting During Labour

Just like nobody has ever taught you how to sleep comfortably – in labour you'll automatically get yourself into the best position to rest. Follow your body's lead.

Positions for Back Labour (Posterior Baby)

Drape your shoulders and chest over the ball and you can move your hips easily. This is a great position for a woman who is having back labour as the birth partner can apply firm counterpressure to mum's back (she'll tell you how much).

All Illustrations © Janelle Durham (www.janelledurham.com)

Water Immersion – The Ahhhh Effect

The bath (or labour pool) is a much underused tool for labour but has significant benefits for mums. If you've every climbed into a warm bath after a stressful day you've experienced the "ahhhh" effect, that feeling you get as you sink down under the deliciously warm water – instantly your mood changes as the warm water releases muscle tension and relaxes you. Women who have access to deep water immersion (labour pools) have the added benefit of a huge boost of oxytocin – shortening their labours while keeping them more comfortable. You are buoyant . . . you feel almost weightless (if you've been feeling like a sumo wrestler for the last few weeks this alone is heaven!) Having experienced the use of a pool during labour I would never give birth without one. Although most maternity units do not currently have labour pools, most would at least have a bath (with the exception of NMH). An inflatable pool to use at home before going to hospital costs a little more than a TENS machine. Women who labour in water have less tears and fewer episiotomies, shorter labours, and it can help speed up a stalled labour as effectively as the drip and mum feels calmer and more in control. A shower can be very helpful too, especially if your partner can direct the spray onto areas where you need it the most (bump or lower back). Although hospital waterbirth is on hold at the moment as hospitals develop their guidelines and policies, there is considerable interest in this option by expectant mums and midwives.

Massage

During some stages of labour, massage can bring welcome relief to the intensity of the contractions. Some women can't bear to have anyone touch them, especially in the late stages of labour. Partners should take the same approach that (hopefully) they have been using throughout the pregnancy, using long, firm strokes following the guidance of your partner.

USING PAIN MANAGEMENT TECHNIQUES

Even with all the planning in the world you will have no way of knowing what your labour will be like or how well you'll cope with it until it starts. Even if you have decided beforehand to have an epidural, you may have to wait a while until you get it, depending on the hospital and where you are in the queue. If your baby decides to come on a Sunday you may not have the option of an epidural.

The best piece of advice you can take is to listen to what your body is trying to tell you. If you feel better standing up, then stand up. If you find massage to be too distracting, ask your birth partner to stop. Pain is the body's way of saying stop! If you sat on the couch and your leg went numb you would automatically move it. In labour you'll do the same; you won't have to think consciously about a list of practised positions, you'll just do what feels good at particular points in labour – and what feels good for a while may not work as the labour progresses. Some mothers feel lots of rectal pressure (in your bum) as the baby moves down. It's usually only momentarily, and it's a very good sign.

GENTLEBIRTH

GentleBirth is a complete antenatal programme that teaches simple but specific self-hypnosis and relaxation techniques for an easier, more gentle birth. A total of 92% of GentleBirth mums polled described early labour as comfortable and active labour as mostly comfortable to uncomfortable.

Hypnosis is not a silver bullet and the techniques take practice. Hypnosis is a skill that you learn and get better at. We believe that having a wide range of comfort strategies is key so you always have options – even if your plan is to have an epidural immediately. With GentleBirth you are learning how to create a labour "toolkit" and understanding how to navigate the Irish system is part of that toolkit. Each couple leaves the class equipped with lots of choices to increase comfort and confidence – including the epidural which is a wonderful tool in itself – especially if you'd had a difficult labour. You get to pick and choose what works best for you on the day – acupressure techniques, the use of hydrotherapy, essential oils, strategies for back labour etc.

The GentleBirth Homestudy program is also available for mums who can't get to a workshop and ongoing support is provided as you work through each week. GentleBirth is definitely not "new age". The GentleBirth program is based on new "edge" science, evidence-based practices and years of research in sports psychology techniques employed by professional athletes. It is the only birth preparation program of it's kind in Ireland.

GentleBirth is not about "training" you to give birth; you innately know how to do that. It's about training your mind to relax so your body can easily do what it was designed for. We haven't lost the ability to give birth instinctively, but we have lost the ability to relax so completely that birth can happen more easily, more quickly and often with significantly reduced pain. How many of us really do any relaxation (both mental and physical) on a daily basis? With GentleBirth, you'll discover that severe pain does not have to be a part of a normal labour.

GentleBirth is perfect for home birth as well as hospital birth. A common misconception for homebirthers is that the pain is necessary. Yes, pain is a great communicator when something is wrong, but in a normal labour pain does not have to be present. Through GentleBirth, you may not feel pain, but you will feel the sensation of tightening or pressure. So although you probably won't feel pain, you will know that labour has started, but in sensations that you choose.

Now I know you're probably sceptical as you read this – I felt the same before I discovered GentleBirth. Even after teaching my first class, in the back of my mind I was thinking, "I hope this works". Then one woman from the class called to tell me her story. She had a birth "show" at 9.00 am, felt fine and went about her day. When she went to her 4.00 pm doctor's appointment he checked her cervix and she had already dilated to 6 cm – and she hadn't felt a thing, other than what she described as "strong Braxton Hicks". For all you first-time mums reading this, generally getting from 1 to 6 cm is very long and can be very painful – no doubt your friends have already shared this with you! This woman went on to birth a few hours later and both baby and mum were very happy – it was her doctor who was in shock! I have heard many more stories such as these. This is not a matter of chance, nor were these particular women easier to hypnotise. Rather, they changed their beliefs about birth through a series of classes, which include developing techniques in visualisation and relaxation.

Today, most of us have already been "hypnotised' to believe that birthing a baby involves many frightening hours of agonising pain. It is something to just "get through" and is rarely an event that we look forward to. All we ever hear is how painful it is, on TV, from family and friends. I bet every other pregnancy/birth book you've read also assumes that birth is intrinsically painful. If this were the case, then it would be so for everyone – and we know it's not. I'm sure you've heard stories of women, maybe even someone you know, who said they didn't even realise they were in labour and gave birth 30 minutes after arriving at the hospital. Remember Laura Shanley's birth story at the beginning of this book? When there is no fear present, labour progresses easily.

GentleBirth doesn't involve being in a trance or a sleep or un-aware of what is going on. Rather, you'll be able to chat and enjoy birth – totally relaxed, but fully in control. You will always be aware of what is happening to you and around you, and never detached from the experience, which is a common misconception especially among medical staff.

Videos of mothers using GentleBirth are incredible, showing labouring mothers awake, alert and in good humour as they ex-perience easy and usually quite short births. In fact, these videos are almost strange to watch; we are just not used to seeing birth as such a relaxed experience.

How Hypnosis Works

If you've ever seen hypnosis on TV or gone to see a stage hypno-tist you may be a little apprehensive and be afraid that you'll end up barking like a dog each time your mobile rings. Well, it's noth-ing like that! Try this little experiment. Close your eyes for a moment and take a deep relaxing breath. Notice the sounds around you which you can hear clearly. Then open your eyes. That's what hypnosis feels like. We go in and out of hypnosis all the time. Have you ever been driving somewhere and were thinking about something else and you miss the turn or you get to your destination and don't even remember half of the drive there – that's hypnosis.

There are so many myths around hypnosis that I'll address just the most common ones here. At no time in hypnosis are you "under a spell" or under the control of anyone other than yourself. You are totally in control and fully awake and aware of everything that's going on around you. You can't get "stuck" in hypnosis. In fact, you are in a trance state right now reading this book – you can hear the sounds around you but you choose to focus on what you are reading.

In the US there has been extensive research into the benefits of hypnosis during pregnancy. The most common benefits are fewer complications (mothers aren't stressed), fewer requests for medication (mothers aren't afraid) and have healthier infants (babies are very relaxed).

Without the presence of adrenaline and stress, your body is naturally filled with endorphins – your own epidural and natural pain reliever. When you're afraid, your adrenaline kicks in and your muscles tighten. Try the following little experiment: make a fist with your right hand as tightly as you can and hold it. After a few minutes your hand will start to feel tired and sore. Now relax your hand – see how much more comfortable that is? Mothers who use GentleBirth don't show the usual signs of labour (panic, fear, pain) and sometimes hospital staff don't believe they are in active labour.

It's important to let your caregiver know that you're using GentleBirth; most hospitals are supportive, but it's always good to let them know in advance. I can't emphasise this enough: GentleBirth is not "pain distraction", and classes do not teach disassociation techniques. Pain is a warning sign that something is wrong and should not be disguised, dissociated from or ignored as is used in traditional hypnotherapy pain "management" techniques.

◇◇◇

Hypnobirthing: Sarah's Story

*H*aving watched my tummy expand, having felt movement where there hadn't been any before, and having gone nine months without having any control over which direction my body was expanding, I knew that I was going to have control over one thing: the birth. No fear and knowing I would be able to control my body when it came to the big day – that's what helped me through the whole pregnancy. To add the icing to the cake was the fact that I had achieved the birth that I had planned and prepared for.

Our first baby, Christopher, swam to the surface of the water birthing pool to meet his long-awaited mommy and daddy. He weighed in at a healthy 8 lbs, 13 oz.

The birth was fantastic and the labour very bearable, all due to HypnoBirthing and having Robert there to put me back on the straight and narrow when all I wanted to do was to climb into bed and go asleep and to be woken up when baby was just about there.

I attended the hospital on the day before Christopher's due date for a routine check-up, wondering whether or not they were going to tell me I had another ten days to go until showtime. To my surprise, I was already 2 cm dilated. I couldn't believe it – I hadn't even felt a thing! Needless to say I was sure it was going to happen that night, but he waited until 4.45 am two days later to make any sign of movement. I had had birth shows from the Wednesday evening all the way up to the early hours of Saturday morning. I woke up having only been to bed two hours before – cleaning the house, rechecking bags, eating pineapple – anything to take my mind off the "When will it happen?" question that was going around in my head. I got a pain across my back that was like a strong period paid. I jumped into the shower and got myself ready, then woke Robert and told him it was time to go.

We rang the hospital midwifery-led unit that I was attending, inform-ing them that I was on the way. They had said not to make my way in until I was getting surges that were 10 minutes apart; according to my timing they were coming nearly every five minutes and lasting about 30 seconds. I relaxed myself and started the HypnoBirthing, thinking of a place that brought back happy memories, imagining how the birth was going to be.

We arrived at the hospital where the midwife led us to the birthing room. I got myself changed and sat on the birthing ball, texting away on my mobile with barely any pains with every surge. The midwife came and did an examination and said that I had reached 5 cm and still had a while to go. We sat in the room laughing and joking, flicking through the television stations. It was very relaxing; lavender oils were burning next to the birthing pool that was waiting to be filled. Throughout the labour I felt warm and drank lots of water, having to make a few trips to the bathroom. When the surges got stronger, I threw up; I knew then that things were progressing further than the midwife had thought.

The pool was filled and I sat into it. The water was lovely; Robert poured it onto my back and talked to me through every surge. We talked about anything and everything, and then put a music CD on to lift the mood. It was still very relaxing; the surges came and went. All that I could think about throughout the labour was that this is how I had imagined it was going to be, and believing that my body was listening to me.

The clock spun on the wall; the time seemed to fly by. Then the urge for baby to birth came. My waters broke around 7.30 am. Christopher's head came out at 8.06 am and finally he emerged fully and swam to the surface at 8.08 am, only 3 hours and 27 minutes from the time I felt the first surge. They had monitored the baby's heart throughout the labour with a doppler and his heart rate had stayed the same. The transition into the world didn't seem to faze him at all. When he arrived he looked up at us, let out a little cry, then lay there quite content. He didn't need to be suctioned at all, and he stayed attached to the placenta until it stopped pulsating.

Throughout the labour Robert talked to me, telling me to breathe the baby down. I got to a stage when the head was coming and I could feel that I was going to tear. It felt to me at that stage as though I had come out of the HypnoBirthing. Robert tried to get me back but all I could feel was a burning sensation. But once the head had come out it was fine; I relaxed again and knew that everything was over and proud of myself *for going through with my plans using HypnoBirthing as my form of pain relief.*

Unfortunately I ended up having a third-degree tear, which I felt none of after the birth. I could walk fine, but I had to go to surgery where I had to get a spinal block and sedatives. This was my worst nightmare, as I hadn't wanted to receive any medical intervention at all. I had had the birth that we had planned and I had achieved it with no medical intervention and with very little pain. I felt terrible after surgery and was annoyed with myself for tearing — but that's life, and I've got passed that.

I felt groggy and disoriented for four or five days. This was perhaps the feeling I would have felt straight after Christopher was born if I had chosen medication as pain relief.

However I had achieved my ultimate birth experience; I had controlled my labour and birth; HypnoBirthing taught me how. My best friend, who had doubted the HypnoBirthing techniques at the start, now thinks it does work; it's all about believing in it and releasing the fear of what others tell you about birth. Robert was in awe of how calm and relaxing the experience was.

I know with the next birth I will do it all over again. Such a wonderful experience, with no fuss or excruciating pain, a natural progression of life, where you are aware of your senses and what's going on around you and that final knowing of what's happening next.

Labour is Good for Babies!

Too often we hear these days that babies shouldn't have to "endure" the trauma of childbirth, or that birth is so stressful that an elective caesarean would be much kinder to your little one. In rare cases, this may be true. However, what it boils down to is that the stress of normal labour is a good stress ("normal" being a labour that isn't induced or speeded up in any way). As the mother labours, her body produces hormones (endorphins) to help her deal with pain. As she does this, her baby's adrenal glands are stimulated and they begin to produce high levels of adrenaline, or stress hormones. This foetal stress response is designed to help the baby make the transition to life outside the uterus.

The activity of birth helps your baby in the following ways:

◊ Helps baby to breathe. The hormones produced help your new-born keep his lungs expanded. As it keeps the lungs open it helps your baby to clear amniotic fluid from his lungs.

◊ Increases blood flow to your baby. Stress hormones help send more blood to the baby's brain, heart and kidneys.

◊ Increases energy supply to the baby. This is what keeps the baby satisfied until breastmilk comes in.

◊ Facilitates bonding. That alertness your newborn has is directly related to these hormones. A more alert baby draws parents in and he or she is more responsive to parents and others.

◊ Increases immunity. White blood cell numbers are increased as he adrenal hormones are secreted.

Studies have shown that while epidural anaesthesia does not affect the levels of stress hormones, there is a significant difference between babies who are born vaginally versus planned caesarean. If a caesarean does become necessary during labour, even early on, the baby has more adrenaline and adapts to life outside the womb quicker than counterparts born via scheduled caesarean prior to the onset of labour. For this reason, some consultants will delay elective caesarean until after the onset of labour when possible.

© Robin Elise Weiss and pregnancy.about.com.
Reproduced with kind permission.

POSITIONS FOR BIRTH

I have never come across a labouring mother who opted to birth in the traditional (on the back) position voluntarily (unless she's had an epidural). Many will end up back on the bed as a result of staff recommendations. As your baby moves down, it has to navigate the tailbone, which will move out of the way once you are not on your back. You're also less likely to get an episiotomy if you choose the position you birth in (the diagram on page 68 illustrates this nicely).

The hands and knees position can be great for back labour (when your baby's back is lying against yours, also known as OP or posterior presentation). You'll find just rocking your pelvis will be very helpful and can help your baby rotate.

If you've had an epidural or a very long tiring labour, birthing on your side with your partner or midwife holding your leg can be helpful. It allows the pelvic bones to expand (but still leaves you vulnerable for an episiotomy).

The supported squat is effective but can be tiring for the birth partner. Your birth partner will stand behind you and "hook" you under the arms with his arms. Benefits include an open pelvis and the advantage of gravity. Mum is free to rotate her hips, helping her baby into a good position for birth.

If you have an epidural or just a tiring labour this position is better than the traditional (flat on your back) position.

All illustrations © Janelle Durham (www.janelledurham.com)

**Birth Partners! How You Can Help Your
Partner during Labour**

Think "PURRRR":

◊ **P**osition: Is your partner changing her position regularly and moving about?

◊ **U**rination: Are you reminding her to go to the bathroom every hour?

◊ **R**elaxation: Is she as relaxed as possible?

◊ **R**espiration: Is she breathing even, relaxing breaths and not gasping?

◊ **R**est: Is she making the most of the break between contractions to rest?

◊ **R**eassurance: Are you giving her constant encouragement and reassurance?

Tips for your Birth Partner on the big day:

◊ Remember to eat and drink

◊ Wear loose, cool clothing

◊ Stay as relaxed as possible

◊ Take a break if you need to.

*© National Childbirth Trust, www.nctpregnancyandbabycare.com.
Reproduced with kind permission.*

Routine Medical Interventions

FAILURE TO PROGRESS OR FAILURE TO WAIT?

Some Irish hospitals strictly follow active management policies to manage your birth. Once you are admitted you are expected to dilate at approximately 1 cm per hour. (Talk about pressure to perform!) Some women will dilate 1 cm and others may not. As you probably know by now, there's no such thing as a textbook pregnancy or birth. There is some evidence to show that the stress and excitement of arriving at the hospital may trigger adrenaline, which is the body's "fight or flight" response and may cause your dilation to slow down or stop for a time. It is at this crucial time when it is critical that your partner reassures you that you're doing great and helps you to relax. The hormones that are present when you conceived are the same ones you need to help you give birth; for most people, having sex in a brightly lit public area with strangers coming in and out of the room and interrupting them wouldn't exactly set the mood!

What Happens If I Don't Dilate Quickly Enough?

If there are no indications of a medical problem, then patience is your best friend. You can ask not to have your labour augmented (speeded up). You can choose not to have your waters broken. You may like to try the more non-invasive method of nipple stimulation or even just a change of position. Nipple stimulation causes a release of oxytocin from the brain, which in turn causes the uterus to contract, and can restart a labour that has slowed down.

No woman is the same, and labour will progress at different rates for everybody – and usually at the right time, all by itself.

When are Medical Interventions Necessary?

Medical interventions are necessary in a medical emergency but when they are routine (i.e. hospital rules) then they can create problems for the 90 per cent of mothers who have normal births. Episiotomy, forceps delivery, continuous **foetal monitoring, ventouse** delivery and amniotomy are all common medical interventions.

Maybe it's just me, but I don't want anything "routinely" done to me that sounds like lobotomy – such as episiotomy or amniotomy. Following are some of the routine procedures "offered" to mothers in Irish hospitals. The important thing to remember is that if it is done routinely then it definitely isn't supported, in the case of normal births, by current research.

AMNIOTOMY (RUPTURING YOUR MEMBRANES)

Some of you reading this will have had your waters artificially released in hospital. For some women this is not a big deal and labour progresses fine. But there are risks associated with this procedure, and very few benefits. I wonder how many of you have had the following experience: your midwife comes to see you and says, "Let me check you and we'll see how far along we are, shall we?" You look at your hubby, who shrugs his shoulders, and you nod. The midwife roots around for a bit, then announces, "About 3 cm. Now I'm just going to pop your waters so we can see how the baby is doing; you won't feel anything, just a gush of warm water." It's all over in seconds. This scenario is played out in many hospitals throughout Ireland on a daily basis. You have just had a medical intervention performed on you that was not agreed to by informed consent. At no time were the risks and benefits of this procedure explained to you, nor were you given an opportunity to ask about alternatives.

As long as the membranes remain intact, the baby and the cord float inside a water balloon. The fluid protects umbilical cord blood vessels from the pressure of contractions. When you remove the fluid early in labour, that protection is gone and the contractions can impede blood flow, causing foetal distress.

Another risk of early **artificial rupturing of membranes (ARM)** is cord prolapse – that is, the cord descends into the birth canal ahead of the baby. This will most likely result in a section. Routine early amniotomy shortens labour by about an hour but also increases caesarean rates. When data from seven trials in which women were randomly assigned and not assigned to early ARM, the women who had an ARM were 20 per cent more likely to have a section. When left alone, the waters usually release when the cervix has dilated to around 7–8 cm; at this point, your baby has had the benefit of being able to move through the pelvis and get into the best position for birth.

Some hospitals prefer to rupture membranes routinely (as soon as you are in labour). This practice is outdated and no longer recommended. The least invasive way to check on your baby's well-being is to listen to the hearbeat. You are carrying precious cargo – the waters act as bubblewrap for your baby in his/her final journey into your arms.

Procedure	Artificial rupture of the bag of waters (Amniotomy)
What is it?	Breaking the amniotic sac surrounding the baby with an amniohook
Who needs it?	When there are other signs of distress there may be a need to see the colour of the amniotic fluid
Who doesn't need it?	Most pregnant women

Procedure	Artificial rupture of the bag of waters (Amniotomy)
Risks	1. Sets "time clock" running for need to deliver your baby

2. Infection

3. Prolapse of umbilical cord if done too early

4. Decrease in pH of newborns with early amniotomy

5. Umbilical cord compression (increase of foetal distress) |
| *Benefit* | Small decrease in labour time |

Source: Janelle Durham (www.janelledurham.com)

EATING IN LABOUR – WHY IT'S GOOD FOR YOU AND YOUR BABY

As pregnant mums you've probably never been more focused on food than any time in your life. Even analogies about baby's size and our body parts are associated with food – as if we weren't obsessed enough. Your baby is the size of a bean . . . your uterus is now the size of a grapefruit . . . your boobs are like . . . (well you get the picture!) You've probably spent endless hours online researching what you can and can't eat during pregnancy.

Some mums have cravings and can't get enough of a particular food, others struggle with all day morning sickness and it takes a huge amount of willpower and determination to even get a few Ritz crackers past your lips.

There's also "pica" which is the term for unusual cravings. The reason that some women develop pica cravings during pregnancy is not known for certain. There is currently no identified cause, but according to the Journal of American Dietetic Association there may be a connection to an iron deficiency.

Some speculate that pica cravings are the body's attempt to obtain vitamins or minerals that are missing from a mum's diet. The most common substances craved during pregnancy are muck/clay. Other pica cravings include burnt matches, stones, charcoal, mothballs, ice, cornstarch, toothpaste, soap, sand, plaster, coffee grounds, baking soda and cigarette ashes.

Science recognises that good nutrition during pregnancy is essential for both mum and baby. Newly pregnant mums often spend a significant amount of time "grazing" or snacking regularly to keep their blood sugar normal.

If you've missed a meal lately you've probably experienced some of the following side effects:

◊ Increased crankiness

◊ You feel exhausted due to low blood sugar

◊ You may even feel faint or pass out.

Skipping meals during pregnancy isn't recommended and you'd never willingly starve yourself during your pregnancy . . . so why would you do it in labour?

Let's look at the history of where this began and what can happen when a mum is refused nourishment during labour (assuming she's hungry – some mums have no interest in eating).

Mendelson's Syndrome is the inhalation of gastric contents and is a risk during intubation for a general anaesthetic (you've probably seen intubation on *Grey's Anatomy*). However most caesareans are performed with a spinal or epidural these days. It is rare to have a general anaesthetic for a caesarean birth. The original article by Mendelson dates back to 1946 so it's a little bit outdated. The great news is that in 1961 a technique called Sellick's manoeuvre was discovered which minimised the risk of gastric contents entering the lungs during a general anaesthetic.

What a breakthrough for labouring mums. It meant that all normal low risk women (80–90% of mums reading this) could go back to eating in labour again! Yay! But wait a minute . . . that was nearly half a century ago . . . obviously some hospitals missed that memo.

Without food for a long period of time a labouring mum's body enters into ketosis. When you first deprive your body of food your metabolism begins to shift to accommodate this. The first stage is known as lipolysis, and means your body is burning fat to provide you with energy (sounds like a great way of burning off those extra pregnancy pounds, after you've had your baby!).

Ketosis is the second part of the process that takes place when your body has no carbs to provide it with energy so it needs to use the energy from the fat being burned. In a nutshell, the unused portions of the fat cells are called ketones, and are removed from the body in the urine. Ketosis is a signal that you are breaking down your fat reserves . . . your body is effectively eating itself to give you energy during labour.

So you're at the hospital, starving, hot, cranky, exhausted – and that's just your partner! Plus you feel pain much more intensely! Not exactly the recipe for a positive birth. Of course, some mums have no interest in eating in labour – if you're very anxious and afraid during labour adrenaline arrests the digestion process. If you're giving birth in a hospital that is stuck back in the 1940s bring along some snacks for yourself and your partner, just in case you do get hungry. Chances are your won't be in the mood for a Big Mac.

Even in these 1940s hospitals there are some fantastic midwives who are happy for you to snack to keep your energy levels up if you're hungry, so all is not lost! On one side of the Liffey you can eat and drink all you want, and on the other side you get a cup of ice chips – YUM! (For once, being a Northsider has it's advantages . . .). For more information on which hospitals support mother-friendly principles and evidence-based international practices have a look at Cuidiu's comprehensive consumer guide listed in the resources section later. Bon appetite !!

Procedure	Policy of NPO (Non Per Os — Latin for Nil by Mouth)
What is it?	Mother is allowed nothing by mouth
Who needs it?	Women who are very ill (a specific medical indication)
Who doesn't need it?	Pregnant women who are not ill
Risks	1. Lack of energy to do the work of labour 2. Dehydration 3. Poor foetal heart rate tracing due to maternal dehydration
Benefit	Reduces the risk of aspiration under general anaesthetic (debatable).

Source: Janelle Durham (www.janelledurham.com)

EPIDURAL

The epidural is the most common way of managing pain in labour (see pages 81–82). The epidural works by injecting a pain medication near particular nerves in the back, blocking these nerves from transmitting pain sensations to the brain. The effect of the epidural is localised to your abdomen, lower back and legs. The anaesthetist will place a sterile drape over your back, and wipe it with an antiseptic solution. You may feel a sting from the injection to freeze the area of your lower back where the epidural needle is being placed. Between contractions, you should only feel pressure as the epidural needle passes between two vertebrae to the epidural space. A thin plastic tube is passed through the needle and the needle is then removed. The remaining flexible tube is taped to your back.

A new development in Irish maternity care is a patient-controlled pump, so that you can receive medication when you need it; this is not available in every hospital.

Is it the Right Choice for You?

Most women who receive an epidural appreciate the respite from pain; they do, however, acknowledge that there are trade-offs involved. You may experience shaking, itchiness and nausea. You'll also need continuous monitoring, an IV and a catheter to drain your urine. A few women get incomplete pain relief or find that it just doesn't work.

The epidural affects your experience of labour, and not always positively. The epidural limits your ability to use a variety of positions to help the baby rotate and descend into the pelvis. However some Midwives (with the help of your partner) can reduce those effects by helping you into an upright position on the bed.

The epidural has many potential side effects – see table below. Did you ever wonder why you can't have an epidural at a home birth? It's because the potential side effects are so risky they couldn't be managed at home.

A rare side effect of the epidural is a severe headache, caused by the epidural needle being inserted too far: instead of stopping in the epidural space, the needle punctures the membrane that surrounds the spinal cord. Sometimes, an injection to "patch" the spot that was pierced by the epidural needle is used to relieve a very bad headache.

Remember that the epidural is only one pain-relieving technique. You will need others to get you through early labour and possibly later labour as well. Even with an epidural, you may experience small windows of pain or a return of pain when it is time to push your baby out. Now is the time to learn and rehearse coping skills. Many women find techniques and good support are all they need to cope with contractions right through to the birth (see pages 92–98). But for those who want more pain relief, or who are unfortunate enough to experience unusually long or complicated labours, the epidural can be a wonderful option.

Birth partners: remember that your job is not over just because mum is physically feeling more comfortable after an epidural. Your partner still needs lots of emotional support and encouragement during this time.

Procedure	Epidural anaesthesia
What is it?	Regional anaesthesia of lower two-thirds of body
Who needs it?	Women who do not have access to comfort measures and are not able to tolerate or don't want to tolerate the pain of labour; some women with high blood pressure
Who doesn't need it?	Women with continuous support and access to a wide variety of comfort measures and maternal positions; women with blood-clotting problems
Risks	1. Decrease in maternal blood pressure 2. Decrease in foetal heart rate 3. Lack of variability in foetal heart rate 4. Mother often needs a catheter (can't feel a full bladder) 5. Increase in chance for urinary infection 6. Itching 7. Prolonged labour 8. Increase in need for instrumental delivery via forceps or vacuum aspiration 9. Reported increase (in some studies) of caesarean section (two to fourfold), especially in first-time mothers 10. Increase in need for episiotomy 11. Headache 12. Respiratory arrest or paralysis in rare cases 13. Increase in labour interventions 14. Infection 15. Ineffective pain relief 16. Increase in maternal temperature 17. Breastfeeding difficulties (babies may be sleepy and have no interest in the breast) 18. Mobility is affected for some time after birth
Benefit	Pain relief when other comfort measures are ineffectual or when a caesarean is needed.

Source: Janelle Durham (www.janelledurham.com)

Monitoring Your Baby

Listening to the baby's heart has been used for many years to gain a sense of how the baby is doing during labour. Initially it was thought that this continuous monitoring would reduce incidents of brain damage to babies because distress could be picked up quickly. Not so. Continuous foetal monitoring was not the silver bullet it was expected to be. Midwives and doctors began to spend more time "mothering the machine" instead of mothering the mother.

There are a variety of ways that you your midwife can check your baby's heart rate – fetoscope (a modified stethoscope), handheld doppler unit and the electronic foetal monitor (CTG). The fetoscope and doppler are used for "intermittent" monitoring, meaning every 15 minutes or so. The CTG is a continuous recording of your baby's heart rate and requires you to stay still (usually lying down) while two transducers record your contractions and your baby's heart rate. The CTG is still used in may Irish hospitals for a 20 minute "admission" trace. This is no longer recommended for healthy women and babies. UK and US guidelines recommend that intermittent monitoring is as effective. Continuous monitoring with a CTG has no additional benefits and in fact has around a 92% false positive rate of distress in unborn babies. With such a high false positive rate you have an excellent chance of ending up with a caesarean if you accept continuous monitoring without a compelling reason (that is, a reason more than "it's policy").

Procedure	Continuous electronic foetal monitoring
What is it?	Continuous electronic tracing of foetal heart rate
Who needs it?	A foetus with intrauterine growth retardation or an ill foetus or a baby considered high risk
Who doesn't need it?	Normal babies, although checking the foetal heart tones periodically is as effective and complies with the American College of Obstetricians and Gynaecologists (ACOG) standards
Risks	1. Increases rate of caesarean section unnecessarily 2. Increases in false diagnosis of foetal distress
Benefit	Constant surveillance of an ill baby.

Source: Janelle Durham (www.janelledurham.com)

EPISIOTOMY

Of all the squeamish discussions about birth experiences, probably nothing makes you cringe and cross your legs quicker than when talk about labour turns to the big E – no, not the epidural, but the episiotomy.

More and more women in Ireland are questioning a once-routine procedure that involves enlarging the opening of the birth canal as the baby's head crowns. Your doctor or midwife makes an incision in the perineum (the tissue between the vagina and anus). Some hospitals continue this outdated procedure despite significant studies that show routine episiotomies cause more harm than good.

First a simple demonstration: if you hold a piece of cloth at two corners and attempt to tear it by pulling at the two ends, it's very difficult to rip. However, if you make a small snip in the centre, and pull the corners the cloth rips easily with no resistance.

According to www.maternitywise.org, those who support the practice, episiotomies have the following benefits:

◊ Speed up the birth

◊ Prevent tearing

◊ Protect against incontinence

◊ Protect against **pelvic floor** relaxation

◊ Heal easier than tears.

The following have been reported as side effects of the episiotomy:

◊ Infection

◊ Increased pain

◊ Increase in third and fourth degree vaginal lacerations (euphemistically called extensions)

◊ Longer healing times

◊ Increased discomfort when intercourse is resumed.

Routine episiotomy (as opposed to episiotomy for an emergency situation such as foetal distress) is a typical example of an obstetrical procedure that still exists despite a total lack of evidence for it and a considerable body of evidence against it. So how can you avoid an unnecessary episiotomy? Some preventative measures that www.maternitywise.org recommend are:

◊ Choose a doctor who doesn't do routine episiotomies. Ask your caregiver how often he/she finds it necessary to do them.

◊ Good nutrition.

◊ Do your Kegels (exercise for your pelvic floor muscles).

◊ Prenatal perineal massage.

◊ Slow controlled pushing instead of directed pushing by doctors and midwives — only push when you feel the urge (see below).

◊ Birth off the bed, not on your back.

Remember, as with any medical procedure, there are always circumstances where episiotomy is a valid and necessary option. The only time most caregivers would agree that an episiotomy is appropriate is when the baby is close to being born and an urgent problem develops.

Episiotomy: Myths and Realities

◊ *Woman is a first-time mother:* Studies that attempt to restrict episiotomy do not find that having a first baby is, in and of itself, a reason for episiotomy (in some Irish hospitals, at least a quarter of first-time mothers are surgically cut).

◊ *Caregiver believes a tear is about to occur:* Performing an episiotomy for this reason has not been shown to have a protective effect and may be counter-productive.

◊ *Belief that episiotomy prevents pelvic floor weakness:* Women are just as likely to have weak pelvic floors or urinary incontinence in the early months after childbirth with or without an episiotomy — caused by the pregnancy, not necessarily the birth. Women with no episiotomy and no or only a tiny tear at birth (intact perineum) have the strongest pelvic floors, while women with tears into the anal muscle have the weakest pelvic floors. Women with spontaneous tears do just as well as, or better than, women with episiotomies.

◊ *Belief that episiotomy is easier to repair (to stitch closed) than a tear:* No research supports this claim. Certainly the tear that occurs when a midline episiotomy extends into the anal muscle is more difficult to repair than a small tear. With optimal care, many women will need no more than a few stitches or no stitches at all.

◊ *Belief that episiotomy heals better:* An episiotomy of either type is more likely to have delayed healing or to become infected in comparison with no episiotomy. A mediolateral episiotomy is more likely to scar and heal pulled to one side compared with the tears that may occur with no episiotomy.

© www.maternitywise.org. Reproduced with kind permission.

Procedure	Episiotomy
What is it?	Surgical incision in the perineal muscles and tissue
Who needs it?	Women whose babies must be delivered immediately due to low heart tones
Who doesn't need it?	Most women in childbirth
Risks	1. Increase in third- and fourth-degree lacerations involving the rectal sphincter 2. Postoperative pain 3. Sexual dysfunction due to long-term perineal pain 4. Infection.
Benefit	Minimal decrease in length of second-stage labour and speeds delivery in a real emergency.

Source: Janelle Durham (*www.janelledurham.com*)

DELAYED CORD CLAMPING

Most Irish mums don't get a lot of information about the third stage of labour – other than "you'll be getting an injection to stop you bleeding". You're probably thinking – "good lord there's a third stage to think about!" It's such an emotionally charged moment when your baby is handed to you that we don't spend much time thinking about what happens immediately after. In Ireland, delayed cord clamping is usually only seen with midwife-led care, community midwives or homebirth and a few short minutes can make a significant difference in getting your baby off to the healthiest start possible. There has been an increasing number of studies published with regards to the timing of cord clamping. In one study the main benefits cited are:

◊ Increased levels of iron (Ireland has high rates of iron deficient anaemia)

◊ Lower risk of anaemia

◊ Fewer transfusions, and

◊ Fewer incidences of intraventricular haemorrhage.

A two-minute delay in cord clamping increased the child's iron reserve by 27-47 mg of iron, which is equivalent to one to two months of an infant's iron requirements. This could help to prevent iron deficiency from developing before six months of age.

A dad once said to me jokingly that isn't it a pity babies aren't born deflated (making for an easier labour) and we just inflate them when they come out. In fact, that's exactly how nature designed the third stage of birth. Up to one-third of your baby's blood stays in the placenta until after your baby is born and then it is pumped into your baby "inflating" him – around 65% of the total blood volume being transfused into your baby happens within the first minute after birth. So if the cord is clamped immediately that blood is left in the placenta and your newborn has been deprived of a significant quantity of blood. The placenta has acted as your baby's life support system for the last nine months, so as your baby is getting used to using his lungs for the very first time it is best that we leave that back up system in place for the most gentle transition possible – even more so if a newborn is having trouble adapting. In the UK, new guidelines are underway for resuscitating babies at the bedside with the cord still attached so the baby is still getting that precious oxygen through the cord even if he is slow to wake up.

Procedure	Immediate Cord Clamping
What is it?	Cord is clamped and cut within minutes of your baby being born
Who needs it?	Only women having a managed third stage who have had syntometrine (synthetic oxytocin) to expel the placenta
Who doesn't need it?	Most pregnant women
Risks	1. Deprives your baby of oxygen; if your baby is having breathing difficulties immediately after birth and the cord is still pulsating, it makes sense to keep the cord intact so the baby has two sources of oxygen as he adjusts to breathing outside the womb 2. Deprives your baby of nutrients through placental blood supply 3. Reduces your baby's total blood volume by approx one-third
Benefit	Minimal decrease in length of second-stage labour and speeds delivery in a real emergency.

Source: Janelle Durham (*www.janelledurham.com*)

OTHER INTERVENTIONS

Sometimes if your caregiver suspects your baby is in distress or if you've had a long labour and are just too exhausted to push, your doctor may need to use a forceps or vacuum to deliver your baby. You're more likely to need some help with the last few pushes if you've had an epidural. The epidural relaxes the pelvic floor, so it doesn't have the resistance that your baby needs to rotate into a good birth position and seems "stuck".

Forceps

Forceps look like metal salad tongs. It comes in two pieces that your doctor will insert into your vagina (you'll never quite look at salad tongs the same way again) and place around the sides of your baby's head. There is a mechanism to fix the forceps once they have been correctly placed so that they don't come apart. Your midwife will probably put her hand on your bump and watch the monitor to see when there is another contraction coming. You'll then be instructed to bear down and push hard with your next contraction as the doctor pulls. You'll most likely be given an episiotomy.

In general, babies born with forceps are fine but can sustain minor bruising to the head and face, so don't be alarmed.

Ventouse

The ventouse is a suction cap made of silicone plastic. It fits onto the baby's head rather like a little cap. Once the cap has been positioned, air is sucked out of it by means of a vacuum device (like a bicycle pump). The doctor then pulls as the mother pushes; just like with the forceps, often a midwife will also be pushing on your bump to move your baby down the birth canal.

Some babies can be quite bruised after a ventouse delivery in the form of a blood blister around the area of the vacuum cap and may develop some jaundice from it. After a long labour your baby may appear quite cone-headed and the blister may accentuate that, but it's usually superficial and doesn't affect your baby's brain. The swelling usually goes down after a few days.

Research suggests that a ventouse delivery is better for mum and baby as there appears to be less damage to the mother's pelvic floor and it is gentler than a forceps delivery. Assisted deliveries can be scary for you, your partner and your baby, so the best advice is to avoid interventions that can directly or indirectly increase your chances of needing them (amniotomy, epidural, birthing on your back).

Directed/Coached Pushing

Another less-known "intervention" which is coming under scrutiny is **directed or coached pushing**. Many researchers now suggest that, once the second stage is reached, a period of rest should be allowed before any vigorous pushing in order to allow the head to descend and rotate slowly, allowing gentle stretching of the tissues and conserving energy. Directed pushing only reduces the birthing time by a few minutes. In an undisturbed natural birth, there is a phenomenon called the **foetal ejection reflex** – in other words, without any active pushing, your body will automatically push the baby out in an uncontrollable reflex action.

From experience, it would appear that the majority of caregivers encourage directed pushing with breath-holding in the second stage (pushing stage) of labour to speed things up. It's unclear why this is so common; most likely because it's just how the hospital has done things for a long time. However, there is now evidence to indicate that encouraged, strenuous pushing may not be the most appropriate means of managing this part of labour.

◊ *Risks for your baby*: Directed pushing causes a rise in blood pressure, followed by a rapid fall which is only relieved on release of the breath. Several studies have found this to be problematic, causing lack of oxygen to the placenta and baby. Conversely, when pushing was spontaneous (only pushing when you feel the urge or, if you have an epidural, only when the monitor shows a contraction starting), using only the abdominal muscles and with slow exhalation, the baby's heart rate tended to either be maintained at baseline levels or, if decelerations occurred, recovered more quickly.

◊ *Risks for mothers*: The fall in blood pressure caused by directed pushing (also known as the valsalva/purple pushing) can cause dizziness and overstraining of the heart. There is also risk of maternal exhaustion. It has also been suggested that early, vigorous pushing may increase the total pushing time. Directed pushing is also associated with more perineal trauma (those nasty tears) and more postpartum perineal and vaginal pain than does delayed, spontaneous pushing. You also may end up with broken veins on your face and bloodshot eyes . . . not exactly the first thing you want your newborn seeing! And wouldn't it be nice for your baby to be born into a room where the first voice he hears is your voice, or at least quiet voices, rather than three people saying PUUUSH?

LEARNING HOW TO PUSH

This second stage of labour, also known as the "pushing stage", is completely out of your control. There's nothing to learn – your body literally just takes over and you couldn't stop it even if you wanted to. Your uterus has grown into one of the most powerful muscles of your body and it will do nearly all of the work for you. A mum in a coma can give birth to her baby. For me, it felt like a massive spasm – my body just pushed without me doing anything.

It helps to understand how it all works. During labour the top of the uterus is starting to get really thick while the bottom of the uterus (the cervix) thins out. When you get the urge to push the top of the uterus has moved down around your baby and starts to squeeze your baby down. The uterus sort of turns into a big tube of toothpaste with the end of the "tube" rolled up to get the toothpaste out.

No doubt you've watched the scenes on *Private Practice* or *One Born Every Minute* of midwives shouting "come on give me one more . . . put your chin to your chest, hold your breath and push into your bum . . . keep it coming . . . keep it coming." All the while mum is purple in the face and has effectively turned off all the oxygen to her baby and to that marvellous muscle. Coached pushing is no longer considered best practice, and yet we still see it in many maternity wards today simply because old habits die hard.

We know that in studies out of the UK mums who followed coached pushing tend to end up with more perineal injury, pelvic floor problems, more bladder injuries, high blood pressure and exhaustion. What about the babies? Babies born to mums who have continued to hold their breath for extended periods get less oxygen, which makes it harder for them to tolerate the last critical minutes of this phase. Even midwives who still follow coached "purple" pushing will tell you to not push as the baby's head begins to emerge. What they mean is don't help the contractions/ surges with any of your own additional pushing – your uterus will keep nudging your baby down regardless. Slow comfortable breaths are important – no special breathing techniques are required. Follow your body's lead. Most mums who aren't coached will take a breath at the peak of the sensation but won't hold their breath for excessive periods – while their midwife encourages and supports her rather than instructs her.

What about a Mum Who Has an Epidural?

Do you need to be taught how to push if you have an epidural and can't feel anything? Surprisingly, in most cases no. Delaying any coached pushing and allowing the baby to descend passively means better outcomes for mums and babies. In one study, 94% of instances of foetal oxygen deprivation lasting two minutes occurred during active pushing. Even though you may not feel anything with the epi, your uterus is still nudging your baby down. And if you're upright with an epidural even better again! Less chance of needing some "help" with a forceps or vacuum.

So What if You Don't Have an Urge to Push Right Away?

This is known as the "rest and be thankful phase" and it just means your body is getting your baby into an optimum position and the uterus is moving down behind your baby. Imagine someone instructing you to go to the bathroom right now and have a bowel movement! Unless you've had the urge to go nothing will happen, but you'll definitely go purple, exhaust yourself and probably get a few piles too!

So rest and be thankful. If you've had an epidural you'll often still feel an increase in pressure (you'll feel it mostly in your bum) so even though you may not have the intense urge to push you can let your body do the work which means you're not exhausting yourself and your baby. Visualisation can be really helpful during this stage – imagine your uterus was an icing bag and your body is gently squeezing the icing down, or if you're in an upright position imagine there is a powerful magnet on the floor and it's drawing your baby down gently.

So back to the title of this section – learning how to push – you don't learn, your body already knows what to do far better than we can imagine!

Cascade of Intervention

Obstetric interventions can be life-saving procedures for women and babies. Technological advances in proven surgical techniques and better anaesthetics have ensured that the 20 per cent of women who need this kind of help receive the best possible care.

Once the natural process of labour and birth has been disturbed, especially if there is no actual medical emergency, there is a significant risk that the unwelcome side effects of the treatment will make further intervention necessary to remedy the problem. This phenomenon is known as the cascade of intervention and is illustrated in the diagram below. It's like the domino effect: once it's started, it has a knock-on effect in your labour and more interventions become necessary.

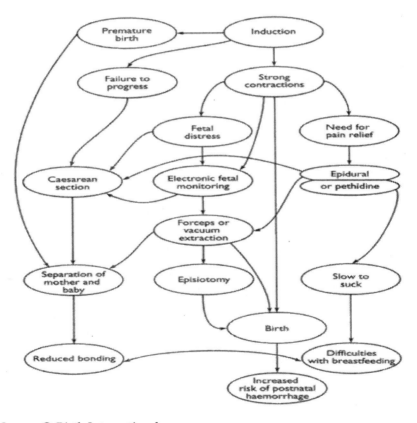

Source: © Birth International

Multiple Births

WHAT IF IT'S TWINS?

The diagnosis of twins can feel like an out-of-body experience for many. You may have suspected that something was up because you've never felt so sick in your life (caused by a sudden increase in hormones), but when you're given the news that there are two or even three heartbeats you may feel like you've just entered the twilight zone. Most consultants consider twin pregnancies high risk, which does not imply that the birth will be a normal, full-term one, but it does mean that the hospital will monitor you more closely. About half of all multiple pregnancies result in premature births (i.e. before week 37), but unless and until that happens to you, focus on being in the half that go the full term.

You will undoubtedly have to see your consultant or midwife more often – probably weekly by the sixth month – and your own health and the babies' progress will be very closely monitored.

Possible Complications

Aside from the chance that your babies will be born prematurely, the most common problems include:

◊ You're going to feel HUGE. Get lots of rest and get help from family and friends. If you've already had a baby, then think of the way you felt when you were nine months' pregnant . . . then back that up to about seven months . . . in other words, two extra months of fat fingers, swollen ankles and sore muscles.

◊ **Pre-eclampsia** develops in about 10 to 20 per cent of women carrying twins

◊ **Placental abruption** is also more common for multiple births. Thankfully this is a very rare complication.

◊ Foetal growth restriction, when one or both twins isn't growing at the proper rate, may cause the babies to be born prematurely or at a low birth weight. About half of pregnancies with more than one baby have this problem.

◊ Twin–twin transfusion syndrome is another rare but serious complication in identical twins. One baby gets too much blood and the other too little. Early detection is critical for twin to win syndrome.

What Happens If I Have One of These Complications?

Once you get to about 36 weeks, the risk of delivering a premature or low-birthweight baby decreases significantly. Before this, any complications may require medications, hospitalisation or bedrest. Educate yourself about the more common risks and complications of a twin pregnancy, while trying not to obsess about the things that can go wrong. There are lots of twin support groups that you can connect with to help you focus on the positives. Familiarise yourself with the warning signs of pre-term labour (e.g. waters breaking before 37 weeks or persistent contractions). Make sure you are eating well and staying well hydrated.

What Happens if I'm Put on Bedrest?

If you go into labour early some caregivers will recommend **bedrest**, depending on their policies, even though no research has proven that bedrest will prevent a pre-term birth.

You're may be reading this thinking, "Wouldn't bedrest be soooo nice . . . start my maternity leave early . . . no more dragging myself out of bed on those dark January mornings . . . I can just roll over and go back to sleep." Bedrest can be excruciatingly boring. Sure, a few days in bed can sometimes be just what the doctor ordered, pregnant or not — but two months of it? Be careful what you wish for.

If you are put on bedrest, find out exactly what that means, because the definition can vary from slightly curtailing your activity to literally not getting out of bed for any reason – and everything in between. Bedrest means something different for every woman depending on what the problem is. The following list from Sidelines, a US-based support group for mums on bed rest, can help you nail down the specifics:

◊ How long will I need to be on bedrest?

◊ Can I get up to use the bathroom?

◊ What position should I rest in?

◊ Can I still do things around the house like washing and cooking?

◊ Can I drive at all?

◊ Can I work at home in bed with a laptop?

◊ Can I lift anything?

◊ How often is it safe to stand?

◊ What about caring for my other children? What can – and what can't – I do?

◊ Are there any exercises I can do while on bedrest?

◊ If I'm prescribed tocolytics (a medication that helps reduce re-term contractions), what do I need to know about it? Are there any side effects?

For tips on surviving bedrest, contact Sidelines.org.

When Things Are Not Going to Plan

BIG BABY SYNDROME

Having a "big" baby is a major fear of women facing childbirth. Babies are bigger and healthier these days, but the majority of mums are also healthier too. Years ago when Irish mothers barely had enough decent nutritious food to eat, a diagnosis of a big baby would be a huge relief, simply because big babies were usually a sign of healthy babies. You don't have to look very far these days to hear very healthy women talking about how their baby has been deemed "big" and they are probably going to have a caesarean because they aren't big enough to give birth. When did we buy into the myth that we are destined to be failures at birth? Other mammals don't seem to have these problems.

CPD? Don't Panic!

A diagnosis of Cephalopelvic Disproportion (CPD) means the baby's head is thought to be too large to pass through the woman's pelvis. In the eighteenth and nineteenth centuries, poor nutrition, rickets and illnesses such as polio caused pelvic anomalies, which resulted in loss of life during childbirth. Indeed initially CPD was the most common reason for carrying out a caesarean. In modern times, however, true CPD is rare, since our general standard of living is so much higher and true CPD is more likely to be caused by pelvic fracture due to road traffic accidents or congenital abnormalities.

Often CPD is implied rather than diagnosed. In cases where labour has failed to progress (or your consultant has "failed to wait") or the baby has become distressed, medical staff commonly assume that this is due to physical inadequacies in the mother rather than looking towards circumstances of the mother's care. These problems frequently occur when CPD is not suspected and there are many other causes such as fear and uncertainty, difficulty adjusting to a medical environment, lack of emotional support and non-continuity of carer.

CPD is also sometimes suspected when the baby's head fails to engage, although both this and failure to progress have proved unreliable indicators.

A woman's degree of motivation to achieve a vaginal delivery along with the level of support she receives are likely to be more influential on the outcome than her pelvic measurements. Even in undisputed cases of CPD, it should still be possible for a mother to go into labour without compromising the safety of her baby. In fact, a period of labour prior to caesarean section is believed to reduce the occurrence of respiratory distress and can therefore be beneficial for the baby.

In any case, CPD is difficult to diagnose accurately, since there are no less than four variables that cannot be measured:

◊ The pelvis is not a fixed, solid structure. During pregnancy and labour, the hormone relaxin softens the ligaments that join the pelvic bones, allowing the pelvis to give and expand. The degree of pelvic expansion achieved will vary from woman to woman and from pregnancy to pregnancy.

◊ Babies' heads are made up of separate bones, which move relative to each other, allowing the baby's head to "mould" and reduce its diameter during passage down the birth canal. No one can predict the capacity of an individual baby's head to mould and, as this is a feature of the normal birth process, should not adversely affect the health and well-being of the baby.

◊ The position that a woman adopts during labour and delivery makes a significant difference to pelvic dimensions. Squatting, for example, can increase pelvic measurements by up to 30 per cent. One of the most common positions in which women give birth, that of being semi-reclined, where the mother's weight is on her coccyx (tail bone), restricts movement of the coccyx, which can severely compromise a below-average pelvis.

◊ The position of the baby can be crucial, and whether its head is well flexed or tilted can mean the difference between an easy delivery and delivery being impossible.

> When a diagnosis of CPD has been made, many people still believe that this constitutes a reason for elective repeat caesarean section in future pregnancies, despite the wealth of evidence to the contrary. Indeed, there have been many documented cases where women have been diagnosed as having CPD and then gone on to deliver vaginally a larger infant than the one that was delivered surgically.
>
> Some women will be able to accept a diagnosis of CPD, perhaps even preferring the caesarean way of birth, whereas others will want to be able to come to their own independent conclusions, and some of these may wish to labour again under more conducive circumstances, to have the chance to give labour their "best shot".
>
> © www.caesarean.org. Reproduced with kind permission.

WHAT IF MY BABY IS BREECH?

If you've just been told that your baby is breech (i.e. your baby's legs or backside are coming first instead of his head), take a deep breath, relax and let's talk about it. If you are still less than 37 weeks pregnant, then the good news is that your baby will most likely turn before labour without you doing anything!

If you are 37 weeks or more, you still have choices. Recent research concluded that caesarean section was the preferred birth option, but this study has been heavily criticised and now has consultants all over the world rethinking their approach to breech births. In Ireland most breech births are via caesarean section but some doctors will help you birth a breech baby.

◇◇◇

Vincent's Breech Birth – First Time Mum

From week 32 my pregnancy became a roller coaster. I was on a business trip in Germany where a guy pushed me against a pole on a train because it was so full and he wanted to get out.

Immediately after the push drops were running down my legs and I was scared it could be my water. But it stopped when I came to the hotel and so I thought it might have been sweat or urine. This business trip was so exhausting for me and so stressful. I had to carry my bags because the airport there had no elevator and there was nobody there to help me so I almost missed my connection flight as I had to run with two bags. It was a nightmare. The next day after this business trip I flew with my husband to Austria (our hometown) to attend an ante-natal class.

I thought I would like to hear everything in my mother tongue so I could remember better when I go into labour. The midwife told me to go to the hospital in Austria before I fly home just to check if my amniotic sac wasn't damaged. I had to stay four days in the hospital in Austria. The amniotic sac was not damaged and the water was not broken, but I had a small amount of fluid. They gave me steroids for my baby's lungs just in case I went into labour. I stayed three more days in Austria and returned then to Dublin on a Sunday.

The next Thursday I had an appointment at my hospital in Dublin (Coombe). I was immediately admitted and they treated me like my waters had broken. After a full week in hospital my consultant, who is German, discharged me because he could read the diagnostics from the Austrian hospital. But I had to come twice a week to the hospital for a CTG on Mondays and Doppler Scan on Thursdays to check my amount of fluid. In week 36 I went on Monday to the CTG and the baby was doing perfectly fine. They always had to call the OB to tell how my baby was doing. So the OB came and looked again at how the baby was lying and said it was still breech and next week we would decide if we could turn the baby or not due to the lack amount of fluid.

I went mad and was a bit loud when I said to her that I would not be going for a c-section. A woman in the waiting room heard me and told me her story that she had a c-section and felt terrible. It was a emergency c-section and she was so upset and felt horrible afterwards. And she said I should look for a Doula and recommended Tracy Donegan from GentleBirth. Thanks to the iPhone I started immediately to send an email to Tracy and she responded not even after 30 minutes. So we were in contact now and I told her my story and asked if she would know a hospital which would do the vaginal breech birth. Tracy was immensely supportive. She told me everything she knew about vaginal breech birth and recommended a forum where they talked about breech positions. I joined this group and was now in contact with midwifes from UK where every woman has the right to choose how she will give birth to a breech baby. So it is very common to have a vaginal breech birth there, but still the doctors do recommend c-sections. Tracy also showed a video to me from a woman who gave birth to a breech baby and she was also a first time mum. All these things motivated me so much that my husband and I made the decision to refuse the c-section. Breech is just another variation of normality. This was my motto. And I was so confident in going for a vaginal breech birth. I knew I could do it. My self-confidence was so strong. And my husband trusted my instincts.

The OB here in Ireland came with terrible horror stories. She really tried to scare me and I think that this is very unfair. Instead of just telling you the risks they try to scare you. But I felt strong and I looked in her eyes and said, "Well, and now tell me all risks about having a cesarean and also the afterwards risk for the baby and the mother." And I think that made my point very clear.

So week 37 started and between week 36 and 37 I drank so much water, relaxed all day long but did researching researching researching and got so much help from Tracy. This week I had on Tuesday the CTG, on Wednesday my scan and on Thursday my appointment with my consultant because he was back from his holidays. I felt good this week. CTG was perfect as usual and my scan was a surprise for everyone. The water was back, fully back, not even on the minimum line. No it was fully back. So I went on Thursday to my appointment totally thrilled. The doctor and I decided to try the turning on the next day at lunch time. He was very positive because the water was back. I told him that we would refuse the c-section and he said that he would totally understand my point, but he would have to go through all risks with me. I told him that I know the risks and also what it would mean to have a disabled child, as I come from a family where three siblings had muscular dystrophy and know exactly what a disabled child would mean. And I also told him that I was not scared and that I was so confident in my decision that I know I can do it. He said that we should first wait for the turning tomorrow and if this didn't not work he would write down for me all risks and it would be my decision. Fair enough. I left the room, emailed my husband that we would try to turn the baby tomorrow and wanted to leave the hospital. I went down the stairs and felt like having to go to the toilet.

And then I felt it. It was like in a movie. In the reception of the hospital my water broke. I wasn't scared at all. I was laughing and said to my baby, "Okay, so you don't want to get turned!" I called my husband. "Hi honey, my water broke. It starts now, can you come to the hospital?" It was 4.00 pm on the 7th of July. I went back to admission and they checked everything. I asked them to contact my consultant because he knew my decision and we would have to go know through all the risks and the refusal of a c-section. My husband arrived and was very calm and happy. The consultant came in and said that this was not the plan, but he smiled as well. He was very sorry that he could not be there in the night because he already had the night shift the night before and was totally wrecked. But the good news was that the doctor who was on this night shift was very experienced in breech birth and there was also a midwife who was also very experienced.

So at 4.20 pm the contractions started. Very soft but they started to come every six minutes. Around 6.00 pm I came to the ward. At 7.30 pm I had contractions every three minutes. I was so hungry that I had to eat something. And I ate a lot. You need energy for the birth so if you are hungry, eat! It was 10.00 pm when the contractions were every two minutes so the midwife checked how much I was dilated and I was 3 centimetres. She asked me if I would like to have any pain killers but I said that I didn't want to have anything. I wanted to be fully there to get the full experience. I was absolutely not scared of what would come next.

The doctor who had the night shift came to the ward and told me how I would have the vaginal breech birth. She knew from my birth plan I would like to choose the position when the pressure waves start. But she told me I had to lie down on my back with the feet in the air and nothing under my bottom. Because I got what I wanted I wasn't complaining. I thought this doctor seemed to be so calm and so relaxed when she talked to me that I trusted her completely. At midnight they brought me to the delivery ward. The midwives were very very nice and they were so excited to support my birth plan as they had never seen a breech birth. They went through my birth plan with me (four pages long) and except for a few little things they told me that they could do everything on it. They asked me again for pain killers or gas but I didn't want anything. So the contractions were every minute and became very intense. I wasn't able to sit and lying is not good. Let gravity work for you.

So I started to walk around, danced a little bit (circled my hips) and breathed deep in and slowly out with a AAAHH or an OOOHH sound. This helps you to breathe much slower out. At 2.00 am the midwife checked again how many centimeters I was dilated and it was still three centimetres but something was really good with my cervix. I think it was very thin or short already. So around 3.00 am the contractions were so intense that I felt the urge to push. But I knew I had to wait until I was fully dilated. They checked me again and here it was. I was 9 centimetres dilated so they called the doctor. My contractions were very intense and I could still only stand on my feet. But my legs were already so tired from all the walking and standing so I started to fall asleep after every contraction for around 20 seconds or so. And I always focused on my baby. I thought all the time that every single contraction will bring me nearer to my baby. My husband was so supportive. He pressed acupressure points on my back and forced me to drink after every contraction so I would not get dehydrated. He also motivated me by saying how strong I was and how proud he was. When I could no longer stand the urge to push because it was so intense the doctor checked how many centimetres I was dilated and said, "Well then let's start and follow your instinct when you need to push." The midwife said to me that I should push into my back. I said I couldn't when I was lying on my back and the doctor allowed me for the first pushes to kneel. I did so and the first pressure wave came and I pushed with all my strength and after three times pushing the little bottom of my baby appeared. Now I had to breathe away the urge to push because they needed me to move on my back as already discussed with the doctor. They helped me and I saw the room was full with all the night shift because everybody wanted to see my special vaginal breech birth. It is so rare that they were all excited. I had absolutely no problem with that. This made me just stronger in showing them that it will go easy and good. I waited for the next pressure wave and as it came I started to push with loud AAAHH's and OOOHH's. This helps you to keep your jaw relaxed. I could feel how the bottom came out followed by the legs. It was amazing.

This feeling made me stronger and I started to push again and I could feel that much more was coming. The doctor didn't pull on the baby. This is very important in giving breech birth. Nobody should pull the baby. Just let it come. She just helped with the arms that they didn't get stuck with the head. This is one risk of a breech birth. But if you have someone who is experienced then they know how to help the baby's arms. Now there was only the head which needed to come out. This is one of the scary moments because you need to wait for the next pressure waves and it feels like an endless time in waiting. The hard thing was that the baby was hanging down and I could feel the weight of the baby. And here it came the next and final pressure wave. With all my strength and a very loud AAAHH I pushed the head out and the doctor grabbed the baby and gave it to my chest. I was crying and so emotional.

It was just unbelievable to hold my little stubborn baby which wanted to come out with the little bottom first. It was a boy and my husband and I were so full of love. Everybody in the room was amazed and thrilled. It was a record time in giving a vaginal breech birth with the first child. That's what they told me. Our little man started to search for my breast after 20 minutes and he drank for fully 25 minutes. The whole experience was so amazing and I never felt more love in my life. We called him Vincent William and he is our love, our world and our happiness. I myself felt so strong and I felt like I can do everything. Vincent is totally healthy. The orthopedic and pediatrician checked him and everything is fine. He is a very good drinker and so nice to Mommy and Daddy. He only cries when we change the nappy and he wakes us up only two times per night. A wonderful little star.

You will hear a lot of horror stories around vaginal breech birth. But think twice. In the past it was just normal in having a vaginal breech birth. And look at all the risks in a natural birth. A cesarean is an operation on your tummy. It is not only risky during the operation there is also a risk after it. The baby can have problems with the lungs, metabolism, breast feeding problems etc. And Mommy can have problems afterwards as well. You will have a scar on your uterus for your lifetime. I am not against caesareans if they are necessary. I just think that a breech position does not always need a cesarean. I know that for a vaginal breech birth you need someone who is experienced. But how can they be experienced when all breech babies are caesarean?

If you feel so confident as I did in having a vaginal breech birth, if you feel that you can do it and it's very deep in your heart and your instinct, if you have absolutely no fear – then fight for having a vaginal breech birth.

A head down baby can also ended up as an emergency c-section. I met five women in one week with a case like this. So every birth is with a risk that something can go wrong. I think we all should choose how we would like to have our birth and the woman's voice should be heard. We are the ones who are giving birth to a child.

Tina-Maria and little Vincent

◇◇

◇◇

Jennifer's Birth Story – Second Baby

The path to Jennifer's birth started at 32 weeks. I had a scan which showed that baby was growing well but that she was breech. This was not great news, particularly as we had been hoping for a home birth. We had had a positive experience of a hospital birth with our son, Pete, now two and a half, using hypnobirthing, so we had been very keen to go for a home birth this time round. While the general advice was that there was still plenty of time for baby to turn, I embarked on the process of actively encouraging her to turn. After about a week, I thought that she had (although in hindsight realised that I would have definitely felt something significant had she rotated), so at my 36 week scan I was surprised to find out that she hadn't. At this appointment, I was alone, as my husband, Ciaran, needed to stay at home to care for our sick son. My consultant matter of factly informed me that if the baby did not turn I "would not pass go" and it would be a section. I asked if I could have a scan the following week and initially she declined but then, probably feeling sorry for me, agreed to one.

Amongst the people I phoned that morning was a friend who was an acupuncturist and he scheduled me in for later that day to start a course of moxa. Over the course of that week I attended for several moxa sessions and spent the week engaging in any activity which would encourage baby to turn, including visualisation, hypnosis, inversions and even hand stands in the pool. After a few days I was convinced that there had been some movement in the direction of transverse. The following week, I sat waiting for the scan, quietly chanting my birth affirmations, with a particular focus on those relating to the baby turning, while I gazed at a well worn picture of a baby in the perfect head down position.

On reflection, I realised that these efforts were like saying the rosary in an effort to induce a miracle, which deep down I knew wasn't going to happen. After about half an hour of waiting, I got my answer, baby was still breech, hadn't moved an inch. I asked the sonographer about the possibility of getting an External Cephalic Version (ECV), and she said that she thought that it could be done, but that I'd need to get an appointment with one of the doctors in order to discuss this. Later that morning I met with the registrar that I was under, and she arranged an appointment with one of the few consultants who conducted this procedure, scheduled for the following Monday, the day before I hit week 38.

In the days leading up to this, I went through a whirlwind of emotions, and had to work through the very real possibility of a section, either as a risk factor from the ECV or as the likely outcome if the ECV was unsuccessful. Over this time I became well informed regarding breech presentation and options regarding delivery. The key facts that I learned regarding breech delivery were that a natural breech birth was best for mother and baby once it proceeded without any augmentation of labour or direct intervention, and that if labour wasn't progressing well that a section was the safest option at this point.

It was a tough couple of days. I got so much support from a range of people, both personal and professional, and that really enabled me to have the strength to work through this process. By the Monday, I was in a space where I had made peace with where baby was at, and had changed one of my affirmations from "baby is in the perfect head down position" to "baby is in the perfect position for being born safely". I went to the hospital with a determination to fight for a natural breech delivery, should the ECV be unsuccessful.

From that Monday the path towards labour changed. The consultant decided against carrying out the ECV as the cord was too close to baby's neck. While my initial reaction was disappointment, it was immediately followed by relief, as it now explained why baby hadn't turned given all my efforts. As I sat up anticipating having to fight my corner, the consultant gave me the option of a natural delivery on the basis of labour progressing well. Both Ciaran and I were in disbelief at this positive outcome, and asked him to write down his recommendations in my file, which he dutifully did, with specific instructions to contact him should he be needed.

I felt calmer than I had in weeks, this all felt right, and so I now focused my energies on preparing for a breech birth. Ironically at my regular appointments at week 38 with my registrar and 39 with my consultant, they both now supported the idea of a natural delivery, which just showed the effect of having a "God consultant" write in my file ... perhaps my rosary chanting had actually worked!

Sunday 28th November ... started to snow, 11.30

I had an early night, as I had a real concern about going into labour in the middle of the night, and the disruption that this would be for Pete. Ciaran came to bed some time after one with a weather report...I wouldn't be going to my osteopath appointment in the morning...what does he know that I don't, I thought, and then he explained that it had started snowing.

I looked out the window and it was a winter wonderland, and the snow was continuing to fall. He joined me in the bed and soon my brain began to race. The energy of both of our brains going into overdrive kept us both awake. You see we live in a small townland, at the bottom of a valley, with steep hills on either side. The roads had been treacherous following snowfall last winter, so being snowbound was a real issue. Shall we relocate to friends near the city in the morning....yes was the definite response.

I struggled with sleeping, my brain going through so many possibilities, while at the same time sending baby a strong message that this was definitely not the time to start arriving as it wasn't safe. Soon after the weather report, I started to feel constipated, not particularly bad, but enough to have me feeling a bit uncomfortable, and contributing to my insomnia. Ciaran eventually gave up trying to sleep and got up to watch some TV. I listened to my hypnosis tracks for a while but for a change they did not induce sleep. I then flicked through some TV and was still awake when Ciaran came back to bed some time later. Despite the thoughts and our concerns, I still had an overall feeling of calmness, and eventually nodded off to sleep.

Monday 29th November

We woke up and yes there was still plenty of snow. We made plans to get ourselves relocated and later that day, having driven up our hill, attached to a tractor as a safety line, we made it to our refuge, where there was only a light dusting of snow. While Ciaran got on with trying to get a bit of a day's work in, Pete and I hung out with his almost 2 year old friend and his mother for the afternoon. It was such a weight off our minds to be in a safe place...and now that we were there, my body felt safe to go into labour, following the visualisations of my ideal birth.

In the weeks coming up to labour, I frequently visualised my ideal birth, and while specific details varied, there were a number of key elements to my ideal birth visualisation. Firstly, I'd know when to go to the hospital, and that we would get to the hospital safely. This generally ran alongside the visualisation of our son, Pete being OK, and happily saying goodbye to us as we went to the hospital. I then pictured a gentle, strong labour, as I

137

knew that baby needed to be delivered by me with as little intervention as possible. I pictured my labour being quite private, that the staff wouldn't know how fast I was progressing ... essentially sneaking up on them by surprise before they could start intervening. I pictured a fast second stage, and finally I pictured walking up to the recovery room, a clear sign that I had not had a section. Amazingly, it all unfolded to plan....

I'll know when to go to the hospital

We sat down to dinner and at around 7.00 pm, just as I was about to have seconds, my waters broke. Ciaran was drawn away from an in-depth discussion with Pete about cheese, to follow me into the bathroom, where we confirmed that yes it was definitely time to get moving.

Our little boy will be OK

I told Pete that it was time for Mammy and Daddy to go to the hospital and that our friends would mind him. We chatted for a few minutes then he gave me a kiss and kissed baby and very soon we were off.

The drive to the hospital was quite surreal. It was a calm drive, there was no panic, no need to rush. I felt mild cramp-like pains every now and again. Checking through my hospital bag in my head I soon realised that I didn't have my mp3 player which contained the "Book of Tracy"...in addition to a selection of music that I had hoped to access...hmm could I go through labour without it...yes....no...yes....no turn around...no...needed to keep moving forward, so we dispatched our friend to bring it in to us.

We arrived at the reception, waiting while the male receptionist finished chatting to someone. "I'm in labour," I informed him. He seemed bemused that I was saying this like I was here for my hair dressers appointment. We were directed to the waiting area for the emergency room. C went to park the car and I sat and waited. Some soaps were on the T.V. There were two people ahead of me. I passed the time snacking on granola bars and water, and taking occasional trips to the toilet. A nurse came out to ask if I was OK to wait. I told her that I was, but checked that she knew that baby was breech. She said that she did.

C. came back with bag and pillows. A few minutes later our "courier" had arrived with my essential mp3 player. After about a half our wait, I was called to be seen, and C. was able to come with me (so much better than our previous hospital experience when partners were not permitted in the emergency room).

I was hooked up to the continuous fetal monitor and was asked to press a button when the baby moved…I pressed it a bit randomly, as it was difficult to distinguish a movement from a surge, and in my previous labour I had been asked to press the same button when I felt a contraction. A midwife put a line in, which I found uncomfortable both physically and psychologically. While she did not explicitly state it, she was essentially carrying out initial preparations for a section. Nurses came in from time to time, concern was expressed that the trace was not indicating much movement, and so was checked by a doctor, who had no concerns and a few minutes later apparently it was all fine. C. had a glance at the trace and didn't see any change in the readings for the duration, so there appeared to be a bit of fuss over nothing. The doctor outlined that we would need to see how the trace was going, that this would be the starting point regarding whether or not we could proceed with a natural delivery. I had an internal exam and was found to be only 1cm dilated yet fully effaced. This felt a bit disappointing but I knew it wouldn't help to focus on the numbers game.

The consultant on call arrived, with the greeting of "hi I'm your consultant handshake"…I struggled to send the body language that I was to be an equal participant in a discussion…despite being hooked up to a machine that goes "bing" and being semi reclined. So, the dialogue went roughly as follows… "So, why do you want to have a natural delivery?"… polite smiles from both of us…polite response by me about it being the ideal for baby and I (given that all would be going well)…no actually a caesarean would be the safest for baby…polite smiles from us both.

"And how many children and you planning to have?" I saw C.'s body rise up in the seat.

"Why do you ask?" I was not in a space for indirect conversations.

"Well essentially if this is your last then a section would be the best option, but if not then a natural birth would be more favourable for a future pregnancy."

Polite smiles – file and box that information and put it high on a shelf.

He then said he'd monitor my progress and we'd see how we go. I stated my preference for a supported squat for the second stage of labour – he interpreted this as me looking to go onto all fours. I smiled nicely (again) and explained how I wanted to use gravity to assist me and that it wouldn't be that different from the lithotomy position. He essentially said, "there there we'll talk about that if you get that far."

He left and a few minutes later C popped out and I took the opportunity to have one last opportunity to indulge my fear of a section. I spoke to baby about how this scared me but that we would do our best to have a natural delivery and that however it turned out, it would be OK. I then put these fears in a box on a similarly high shelf, as I went back to focusing on my birth story, with a particular focus of walking up to the ward after delivery.

A gentle, strong labour . . . sneaking up on them by surprise

We ended up being brought to the induction room at around 9.15, as this would be a place where I could be until labour "started to progress." It was a room with three others, where over the hum of machines there was the sound of one woman whimpering in the bed beside me. The time initially passed with answering standard questions, chatting with Ciaran and snacking. Ciaran popped out to get a coffee, a chance that he needed to make the most of whilst I was happy for him to leave. On several occasions I was asked to, "Let us know when the pains get stronger," and I was sporadically given traces while I listened to some vocal music on my mp3 player. From 10.30 or so I found that the surges slowly became more intense, and that I was experiencing them as pain and discomfort. I found that I was drawn to images of water, of surfing the waves, but that, not being very good at it, I kept falling off the surfboard and getting washed over by a huge strong wave. The waves came in patterns of two, one wave which reached a high peak, the second a lower wave, but staying high longer. These waves I experienced as pain, initially breathing through them, focusing on keeping my body relaxed, opening hands, and moving them in swim-like motion, while actively focusing on my jaw relaxing as I breathed out. I found that I was most comfortable sitting on a chair, with my head on the side of the bed, propped up by some pillows. Having my feet flat on the floor felt quite grounding.

Around 11.00 or so, the pain intensified, surges becoming more frequent and stronger. I felt like I was climbing a cliff, nearly at the top, but struggling to get my hand to the last hand hold, and after a few struggles, would eventually get there, but never being sure if I could reach. Around 11.15 shiny shoes were spotted under the curtain, and the consultant stuck his head in… Are the pains getting stronger? Yes, I smiled politely before going back to my body.

Since we had arrived in the induction room I had made several trips to the toilet, and each time the trip became more arduous and resulted in more of my waters releasing. On this particular trip to the bathroom, I had a bowel movement, a sign, I knew, that things were progressing fast, a point of no return. Ciaran was waiting for me outside the door as I tried to time standing up and walking back to the bed before the next surge.

My voice became the outlet for my pain. What had started as a barely audible out breath became a sigh, then a meditative "aw", which then progressed to an animal like call. I found myself drawn to images of a wolf, as the surges became excruciatingly painful, and piling on top of each other. I started to make repeated sounds but then felt a sense of hyperventilation so focused on sustaining the primal sound coming out of my body. As the sounds coming from me intensified, I could feel baby getting lower in my body, feeling an urge to push but knowing that it was too soon. I gripped at and bit into the pillows in front of me. "Baby, we love you," I sang.

I knew that I needed to experience a strong labour and had actively visualised this, and know found myself thinking, "and I wanted this!" I felt that I couldn't go on, and I asked C. to tell me that I could do this. C. kept on reassuring me with what I needed to hear, with a mantra of you *can do this, your body knows what to do. I sobbed to baby to give me a moment's break...baby had other ideas.*

As the midwives quickly realised that labour was progressing fast they wanted to continuously monitor me again, so they struggled to put the monitor around my waist, my body writhing like a caged animal as I lived through the surges. It didn't take long for them to decide that I needed to go into the labour ward. I told them I couldn't walk, as the surges were coming so close together, so they helped me onto a wheelchair as more of my waters released. I have a vivid image of being pushed along the corridor to the labour ward while gripping the chair with all my might, and making a lot of noise. I could feel the sensation of a refreshing breeze from the air passing my face. I bemusedly wondered how wild I must be appearing at this point and that there couldn't have been anyone in the labour wing who didn't hear me.

We got into the labour ward.

There was some mention of a gown, which I dismissed as I started to pull off the remaining clothes that I was wearing in response to a burning heat throughout my body. I climbed up on the bed and kneeled, facing the head of the bed, holding the top bed rail with all my might. Time for another trace, and this time an internal exam. In between surges I negotiated being able to stay in a supported squat or delivering the baby and the Registrar agreed to this, suggested weight bearing on the stirrups with my arms. Back to facing the head of the bed, lots of shouting in the background, yet over that, and my constant "ah" I focused on C.'s voice as he continued to keep me assured that I was doing OK. Another check, an anterior lip, damn. I called to my body and baby to, "open" which I heard distantly echoed by one of the midwives.

I distinctly remember that Ciaran was the first person who told me to start to push, followed by a blurry chorus by others in the room. I now faced them, in a supported squat. Over the next 10 minutes or so, baby was delivered in three pushes. Given that during this time I was just focusing on staying alive and pushing, Ciaran told me afterwards how she came out. First push, out came the bottom and legs, second push out as far as her neck, which had the appearance of being very long. At this point, the Registrar rotated her body about 90 degrees and on the third push her head came out. The cord was quickly cut as she was immediately brought over to the baby doctor to be checked out ... a few seconds later and a loud cry.

We did it, a little girl born at 00.59 on 30th November, her due date ... a natural breech delivery ... and yet all I could say was, "Am I alive?" My body was in shock, and while I never thought I was going to die, I did think that I might break with the pain. In contrast, the nurses and Registrar were busy congratulating me and celebrating how well I had done.

Our little girl, Jennifer, was placed on me soon afterwards, and I held her as they proceeded to manage the third stage. I was then given stitches, I had torn again, unsurprising as I had torn during my first labour. The stitching felt like it took forever ... was she darning a quilt? Eventually the poking and prodding was stopped and our little girl latched on strongly and started to feed ... our beautiful little upside down girl.

I will walk up to the recovery room

... and that is exactly what I did.

<><><><><><><><><><><><><><><><><><><><><><><><><><><><><><><><><><>

Breech Birth: What Are Your Options?

If you decide to choose a caesarean birth consider waiting until labour begins as this will eliminate the risk of prematurity and give your baby the benefits of the labour contractions which are important to prepare your baby's lungs to breathe on their own. Get support. Ask your hospital for their most skilled breech Midwives and consultants and consider the option of an **ECV (manual turning of baby)** this option is recommended internationally and has very few risks. Hypnosis and acupuncture can also be helpful. If you are considering a breech vaginal birth there is a great online documentary called "A Breech in the System" – about one first time mum's journey to her vaginal breech birth.

External Cephalic Version

Research indicates that manually manipulating the baby into a better position is often successful for turning breech babies if done around 38–39 weeks. You will need to find a caregiver skilled in this procedure, and you will need to take a drug to relax the muscles of the uterus while it is being done. As there is always a very slight risk that the cord will become entangled or the placenta start to separate as the baby is turned, external cephalic version should always be done in a hospital, where a caesarean section is available in the unlikely event of such an emergency.

ECV is not pleasant. It's not exactly a gentle manipulation; some force is required by your consultant and probably a midwife. Even after an ECV, some babies will still flip back to a breech position, although it's less likely when done at 38 weeks due to the size of the baby. If, after trying everything, the baby does not move into a head-down position, there may be a good reason why he prefers to remain in the breech position; perhaps the placenta is positioned low down, limiting the space for the baby's head in the lower part of the uterus, or the uterus itself is shaped unusually and is restricting his movements. If the baby does not turn easily, then it must be assumed that he needs to stay where he is (babies are smarter than we think).

"Moxa"

A very successful "do it yourself" technique with a proven high success rate is to use locally applied heat treatment.

The heat from burning moxa sticks – called "moxibustion" – can be used to stimulate the baby's movements and encourage it to turn. These sticks, shaped like cigars, are available from herbalists, Chinese medicine stockists and some acupuncturists (who use moxa sticks for other purposes) and they contain tightly rolled dried leaves of the mugwort plant. They are very inexpensive and two sticks will be needed — they can be used several times.

A randomised controlled trial indicates that approximately 70 per cent of breech babies will turn using this method.

Hypnosis

Although hypnosis is usually associated with giving up cigarettes or losing weight, one of the most interesting new areas of study is the effect it has on babies in a breech presentation in utero. Hypnosis is very effective in changing the position of a breech baby, persuading it to turn, often within minutes of the session. A study on breech babies turned with hypnosis, also showed that these babies stayed in the proper position, where babies turned manually often returned to the breech position.

This ability for the baby to be influenced by the mother's thoughts and suggestions give us even more evidence that we are in communication with our babies throughout our pregnancies. Acupuncture is another option worth trying.

What If My Baby Is in the Posterior Position?

If you are told your baby is "posterior", this means he is facing your tummy instead of your backside; i.e. your baby's back is against yours. Mothers of babies in the "posterior" position can (but not always) end up with long and painful "back" labours as the baby usually has to turn all the way round to facing the back in order to be born. If you're having back labour, then the last place you will want to be is on your back. You'll instinctively get on all fours or into a position that helps your baby rotate into a better position.

You may be able to reduce the likelihood of a posterior presentation by being aware of your posture during pregnancy. There are also "tricks" for turning posterior babies, if yours seems stubborn. These are not evidence-based – just recommendations from mothers who had posterior births on what worked for them.

Tips for Turning a Posterior Baby Before Labour

Avoid positions that encourage your baby to face your tummy. The main culprits are said to be lolling back in armchairs, sitting in car seats where you are leaning back, or anything where your knees are higher than your pelvis.

◊ The best way to do this is to spend lots of time kneeling upright, or sitting upright, or on hands and knees. When you sit on a chair, make sure your knees are lower than your pelvis, and your trunk should be tilted slightly forwards.

◊ Watch TV while kneeling on the floor, over a beanbag or cushions, or sit on a dining chair. Try sitting on a dining chair facing (leaning on) the back as well.

◊ Use yoga positions while resting, reading or watching TV – for example, tailor pose (sitting with your back upright and soles of the feet together, knees out to the sides)

◊ Sit on a wedge cushion in the car, so that your pelvis is tilted forwards. Keep the seat back upright.

◊ Don't cross your legs! This reduces the space at the front of the pelvis, and opens it up at the back. For good positioning, the baby needs to have lots of space at the front.

◊ Don't put your feet up! Lying back with your feet up encourages posterior presentation.

◊ Sleep on your side, not on your back.

◊ Avoid deep squatting, which opens up the pelvis and encourages the baby to move down, until you know he/she is the right way round. Jean Sutton recommends squatting on a low stool instead, and keeping your spine upright, not leaning forwards.

◊ Swimming with your belly downwards is said to be very good for positioning babies – not backstroke, but lots of breaststroke and front crawl. Breaststroke in particular is thought to help with good positioning, because all those leg movements help open your pelvis and settle the baby downwards.

◊   A birth ball can encourage good positioning, both before and during labour.

◊   Various exercises done on all fours can help, e.g. wiggling your hips from side to side, or arching your back like a cat, followed by dropping the spine down. This is described in more detail in an article on www.wellmother.org – "Exercise for relieving backache" by Suzanne Yates.

© www.homebirth.org. Reproduced with kind permission.

Caesarean Section

Please Read Me!

Don't skip this chapter and assume it won't happen to you. Caesarean rates in Ireland continue to rise – currently around 30%. One in three mums will have a surgical birth. It's human nature to think that it won't happen to you but I would urge you to read this chapter. Reasons cited for the rise include more high risk mums, better detection of foetal distress and bigger babies, but a paper published recently by the Economic and Social Research Institute found that "at least half of the rise in c-section rates is due to 'changes in physician behaviour' not older mothers or other risk factors."

When Is It Necessary?

Much depends on whether your consultant (or midwife) follows a policy of active management or expectant management; an active management policy is more likely result in a caesarean. Caesareans will almost certainly be performed in the following cases:

◊ *Transverse lie:* Your baby is lying sideways.

◊ *True CPD*: True **cephalopelvic disproportion (CPD)** occurs when a baby's head or body is too large to fit through the mother's pelvis. True CPD is very rare, but many cases of "failure to progress" labour are given this diagnosis. When an accurate diagnosis of CPD has been made, the safest type of delivery for mother and baby is a caesarean delivery. The problem is, true CPD cannot be diagnosed until during labour.

◊ *Placenta previa*: When the placenta is blocking the cervical opening. A complete **placenta previa** (i.e. when the placenta is completely blocking the opening) in late pregnancy would automatically mean a c-section and maybe even a few weeks of bedrest beforehand. It's quite normal to have some kind of previa midpregnancy, but the placenta usually moves up as the uterus grows. In other words, it will normally self correct – no need for you to do anything.

◊ *Prolapsed cord* (i.e. when the cord comes out before your baby) in the first stage of labour.

Other reasons given for caesareans (usually by consultants with an active management philosophy) but which may not be absolutely necessary include:

◊ *Relative CPD*: That is, when the baby is malpositioned, such as a posterior baby (baby is lying with its back to your back). This can make for a longer and more painful labour. In order to avoid a caesarean, there are ways to help your baby get into the best position for birth (see pages 146–147). Also, avoiding artificial rupture of membranes is important so the baby can make its way through the pelvis with the cushioning of the amniotic fluid.

◊ *Foetal Distress*: This is an indicator that your baby may not be doing well in labour. Foetal distress is very subjective and is usually diagnosed with electronic foetal monitoring. In Ireland, some consultants will take a sample of blood from your baby's scalp to see if your baby is truly being deprived of oxygen. Sometimes just changing position can help. Foetal distress is more common in labours that are induced or augmented with syntocinon.

◊ *Dystocia of Labour (Failure to Progress):* This diagnosis is usually made by an active management consultant, and basically means that your time is up; with an expectant management consultant as long as mum and baby are doing well the labour would continue.

◊ *Maternal Exhaustion*: When a mother has been labouring for a long time and is exhausted before the pushing stage.

WHAT NORMALLY HAPPENS DURING A CAESAREAN?

If you don't have an epidural already you'll be taken to theatre where an anaesthetist will inject the epidural into your back via a thin catheter. You may have some stinging while the area of your back is numbed so the epidural or spinal injection can be inserted but this is usually momentary. You may have some shivering which can result both from the anaesthesia and stress. A catheter will be inserted into your bladder to drain your urine; this is done after the epidural has taken effect, so you won't feel anything. These days it's quite normal for partners to be present during a caesarean, provided you have an epidural and don't need a general anaesthetic, which is rare. Check hospital policy on this.

You will be put on an IV containing fluid and, possibly, drugs. You will probably also be put on oxygen. However, if the epidural doesn't work, you'll be knocked out with a general anaesthetic. If you are just under local anaesthetic, a little "curtain" will be hung below your neck so you don't have to look at the surgery. Sometimes it is possible to see the surgery in the mirrored overhead lights. If you can see anything, try to focus on something else. Birth partners: help keep mum positive and focus on the fact that you'll be meeting your little one soon.

Your pubic hair is shaved where the incision will be, horizontally, just above the pubic bone. You'll probably hear lots of odd noises like the suction machine. Birth partners: stay as calm as you can and focus on your partner's face, especially if blood makes you queasy.

You may feel intense pulling and tugging to dislodge the baby's head from the pelvis. If your baby is in the head-down position (**vertex**), your baby is pulled by the neck backwards out of the pelvis (sometimes with forceps) and then by the head through the incision in the uterus (it's quite small). The baby's nose and mouth are then suctioned to remove any amniotic fluid, mucous and/or meconium from the airway. The remainder of the baby's body is pulled from your uterus through the incision, taking care not to tear the uterine or abdominal incision wider.

Your baby will be checked over while you are being stitched. The umbilical cord is clamped and cut immediately and your baby will be dried off and weighed. Syntocinon/Pitocin is immediately injected into the mother's IV to begin contractions of the uterus to aid in the removal of the placenta. The placenta is removed and examined to ensure all pieces are intact. The uterus is then removed from your body and placed on your stomach for the incision repair. One set of stitches is made in the wall of the uterus, then a second layer of stitches in the outer lining. The uterus is then pushed back through the abdominal incision and into your body. The doctor will count the sponges and gauze to ensure none are left inside you. The abdominal cavity is washed out with water to flush out any bacteria (to prevent infection) and check for bleeding. Your abdomen is then stitched and you are then moved to the recovery area. From the time of the epidural, you should see your baby in about 10 minutes, but the stitching up takes an additional 30–40 minutes.

Within 24 hours, the urine catheter is removed and you are allowed to stand and perhaps walk to the bathroom or shower, but you probably won't want to. Within five days you'll be discharged, with a check of the incision in two weeks. If you think the scar may be infected you'll need antibiotics. Incision pain may occur constantly or intermittently for up to a year.

(*Source*: International Caesarean Network)

Breastfeeding is not impossible after a caesarean but can be more difficult. Try to get your baby on the breast as soon as you get to recovery, provided your baby is doing OK. Some hospitals insist on taking the baby to the nursery after a caesarean birth but you can request that your baby stay with you in recovery if he is doing well. Ask to see a **lactation consultant**. Side-lying to breastfeed will make initial breastfeeding easier. Probably the hardest part of breastfeeding after a caesarean is just getting out of bed to get your baby. Ask the midwife to bring your baby to you as often as you need to nurse him or have someone stay with you as much as possible during the first few days at the hospital to help pass the baby to you. Surgery can affect how quickly your milk comes in too, so don't be surprised if your milk takes a little longer to come in after a caesarean. (It's usually two or three days for a normal birth.)

Risks of Caesarean Section

Risks for the mother include the following:

◊ Infection: The uterus or nearby pelvic organs such as the bladder or kidneys can become infected.

◊ Increased blood loss: Blood loss on average is about twice as much with caesarean birth as with vaginal birth. However, blood transfusions are rarely needed during a caesarean.

◊ Decreased bowel function: The bowel sometimes slows down for several days after surgery, resulting in distention, bloating and discomfort.

◊ Respiratory complications: General anaesthesia can sometimes lead to pneumonia (general anaesthesia use is rare for a caesarean)

◊ Longer hospital stay and recovery time: Five days in the hospital is the common length of stay, whereas it is less than one to three days for a vaginal birth.

◊ Reactions to anaesthesia: The mother's health could be endangered by unexpected responses (such as blood pressure that drops quickly) to anaesthesia or other medications during the surgery.

◊ Risk of additional surgeries, for example, hysterectomy, bladder repair, etc.

In caesarean birth, the possible risks to the baby include the following:

◊ Premature birth: If the due date was not accurately calculated, the baby could be delivered too early.

◊ Breathing problems: Babies born by caesarean are more likely to develop breathing problems (normal labour is good for babies!)

◊ Low Apgar scores: Babies born by caesarean sometimes have low Apgar scores. The low score can be an effect of the anaesthesia and caesarean birth, or the baby may have been in distress to begin with. Or perhaps the baby was not stimulated as he or she would have been by vaginal birth.

◊ Foetal injury: Although rare, the surgeon can accidentally nick the baby while making the incision.

IMMEDIATE CARE AFTER A CAESAREAN

A caesarean section is a major operation, and it is going to take some time to recovery from one. You will therefore probably be kept in hospital for longer than you would if you had had a normal vaginal birth, and you will need more care from nurses and others. You will be encouraged to gently begin to get active; moving around reduces the risk of infection and prevents clots. Either later the same day or the next morning, it is a good idea to get out of bed and sit out for a time.

You will need some help in the first few days; staff are often busy, but do not be afraid to ask.

Tips for Recovery After a Caesarean

◊ Take it slowly. You'll probably feel like you've been hit by a bus the next day. Go easy on yourself. Just getting out of bed is going to be very painful. The midwives will want you up and about quickly; they're not doing it for kicks — it's important for you to be up and mobile to prevent blood clots. Those first few steps are going to be painful and you will need help. If you've never had surgery before, it can be a shock how your body reacts and how much it takes out of you. Take baby steps and don't rush yourself.

◊ Take your pain medications. Even if you are breastfeeding, your doctors and nurses will still urge you to take your medications. You'll feel better and you'll be more motivated to keep up the breastfeeding. The actual amount of medications that will reach your breastmilk and your baby are minimal and quite safe but be sure that your caregiver knows that you are breastfeeding. You will need those medications to help you during those first few weeks in order to walk, sleep, etc.

◊ Let others help you. Swallow your pride and let your partner, family or friends help you with the house and caring for the baby. Even a simple task like climbing into bed can make you feel like a 90-year-old.

◊ Keep your necessities close. Having necessary items such as nappies, wipes, tissues, mobile phone, paper towels, remote control, pain medications, bottles, nipple cream, etc. close at hand will help tremendously. Having them next to you will help keep you from having to continuously get up and down or move from room to room.

◊ Pulling to a sitting position. Those tummy muscles that you once took for granted will be of no use to you for the first few weeks following your operation. To pull yourself from a lying position to a sitting one, be sure to either have someone help you or use something like the back of the couch to pull yourself up gently. Another good trick if you are lying on a couch or bed is to try gently rolling off it (assuming it is not too high off the ground) to the floor and then pull yourself up using a sturdy object such as a table or a nightstand.

◊ Avoid stairs. If at all possible; avoid climbing stairs for at least the first week. If your room is upstairs, set up camp downstairs on the couch.

◊ Create a pillow splint. Laughing, sneezing, coughing or taking deep breaths those first few days will be extremely painful. If you need to do any of those things, take a soft pillow and press it gently to your abdomen.

◊ Avoid greasy foods and carbonated drinks: Once your bowels begin working properly after surgery, you will be extremely gassy.

Gas bubbles will wreak havoc on your sensitive insides. Be sure to avoid anything that will only irritate your bowels further.

◊ Keep checking your incision: You might not want to look at it, but keep a constant check on your incision. Your doctor will advise you on what he/she would like you to do to keep the area clean. Report any inflammation, redness or discharge.

◊ Talk about your feelings: Depending on the circumstances of your caesarean section, you will most likely have conflicting emotions surrounding the event. Top it off with the normal post-partum blues and you may feel like an emotional wreck. Talk to someone you trust about how you feel, or talk with other mothers who have experienced the same things. Don't be afraid to cry and don't feel ashamed of your feelings. It is normal to feel angry, regretful or sad about having a caesarean.

© Jaime Warren and www.caesareanbirth.com.
Adapted and reproduced with kind permission.

CHOOSING A CAESAREAN

More and more women are requesting caesareans in Ireland, and indeed worldwide. The reasons behind these requests include fear of vaginal birth, often after a traumatic first birth; misinformation on the risks of caesareans; and, for some, it offers a sense of control. Caesareans save lives but have become routine "procedures". The risks are well documented. It is major surgery and although it may provide a quick and relatively pain-free birth, the recovery time is often 6–8 weeks and there is an increase in complications for both mum and baby. Some choose caesareans mistakenly thinking that they are avoiding pelvic floor damage but this is often due to lifestyle and the pregnancy itself, not the birth.

A Positive Caesarean

In the UK Professor Nick Fisk has started what he calls a "natural caesarean". This groundbreaking approach to surgical delivery – Fisk calls it a **"skin-to-skin caesarean"** or "walking the baby out" – has been pioneered by him partly in response to the rising caesarean rate. As Fisk started to examine the conventions of surgical delivery, he was struck by how easily they could be challenged. Why, for example, did they need to be done so quickly, when slowing them down would give the parents more chance to participate in their child's delivery and might give the baby a gentler experience of coming into the world? Why, too, was it so important for the parents to be screened off from the mother's abdomen? And was it really essential for the baby to be whisked off for an immediate medical examination, rather than delivered into the arms of his mother?

This is the birth of your child, a completely different surgical experience than any other, an experience to be treated as similarly to a vaginal birth experience as is humanly possible.

If you do need a caesarean, then it would be better for you to receive a spinal/epidural anaesthetic and remain conscious during the operation, participating in the birth of your child.

If an emergency caesarean is necessary under general anaesthetic, then be sure your baby is given to your partner as soon as possible after birth and held by him (hopefully next to his naked chest – skin-to-skin contact) until you are awake and can be told of the baby's sex and well-being (by your partner).

If an elective caesarean is necessary, then you should request that you be able to begin labour naturally before the caesarean is done. That is, you do not want a date and time preset; you wish for your baby to decide the day on which it is ready to be born to avoid any problems with prematurity and for both of you to reap the benefits of your hormones.

Your baby should remain with you at all times – no disappearing off to the nursery with your partner. No matter how "nice" this is, it can affect your bonding with your new baby. If your baby must go to the nursery, then do send your partner and encourage the "skin-to-skin" contact mentioned before. Your baby will really be craving this contact, and he will most likely recognise your partner's voice.

Make sure theatre staff realise that you would appreciate a verbal description of the birth as it occurs. You may have previously felt left out of your past caesarean(s) as your body and labour might have been discussed as though you weren't there.

How about asking the surgeon to leave the umbilical cord long and allow the father or mother the chance to cut it? That way the parents do not miss out on the sensation or their own right to tell their story of "cutting a cord".

Would you like to meet your new baby in his/her unclothed, naked newborn state – a wet, slippery baby? Then request that the baby please be placed on your chest with a warm blanket over you both. It would do a lot to make this surgical delivery a bit more natural for mother, father and baby. And it may even resolve a few inner conflicts that are faced after the birth.

How about breastfeeding your baby straight away? Let them know that you would like to feed your baby while you are being sutured, if you feel up to it, and you would like your baby to stay with you throughout the surgery and even during the recovery. Or you could arrange for the lactation consultant of the hospital (or your own private one) to be present at the caesarean birth and bring the baby to you in recovery, to breastfeed within that first hour of birth.

Let them know that your partner would be delighted to hold his/her child within your view throughout these procedures, if you feel unable to participate in the bonding (at least you would be able to witness it this time).

You may also be able to organise with your doctor to allow a quiet relaxation CD to be played throughout the birth. Don't let it intrude on the birth, though; just enough to gently enhance the experience.

What about that placenta? Most women who birth vaginally get to see it, at least, and maybe you would like to.

Make a birth plan! Have several copies with you and give it to everyone involved in your caesarean! They won't know what is important to you unless you let them know.

Write to the Head of Obstetrics in the hospital about your birth plan. That way, they have plenty of time to fully understand what you want, as well as give them the opportunity to raise with you any concerns they may have. Once you have both reached an agreement about your caesarean then get that agreement in writing and take it with you to the hospital so staff do not have to run around and "get approval" from the appropriate person.

Ask the hospital to take you through every step of the procedure. Make sure they explain to you every light and every sound. Much of the anxiety happens when you can see flashing lights and disturbing noises and you don't know what it means.

Make sure that there is someone to take digital photos of the birth and the baby (in case you are having a general anaesthetic). Then if the baby has to be taken away for observation you can see pictures of the baby as soon as you wake from the procedure. You can use a camera phone but the quality won't be as good — but you can send it to friends and family immediately.

After being wheeled into the recovery room, ask that they dim the lights for you and your baby. (This might not be possible, especially if you have a few other patients in the recovery ward and checks requiring observations are being done all the time).

You might want a special blanket to wrap baby in while waiting with you at recovery. Note that if your baby is with you at recovery, most hospitals will require a midwife to be in attendance. This is why it's a good idea to get the head of maternity and operating theatre involved very early, to assist with staffing requirements.

© www.birthrites.org. Reproduced with kind permission.

Caesarean Birth Plan

This birth plan is intended to express the preference and desires we have for the birth of our baby during a planned caesarean. It is not intended to be a script. We fully realise that situations may arise such that our plan cannot and should not be followed. However, we hope that, barring any extenuating circumstances, you will be able to keep us informed and aware of our options. Thank you.

The Surgery

◊ Spinal/epidural anaesthesia

◊ No pre-operative medications

◊ Partner to be present at all times

◊ Video/pictures taken (my partner can do this)

◊ Partner to cut the cord

◊ Breastfeeding in recovery room

◊ Mirror to view the birth or lower screen.

◊ Postpartum and Baby Care

◊ Breastfeeding only

◊ No pacifiers or glucose water

◊ No separation of mother and baby

◊ Paediatric exams in the mother's room

◊ Do not bathe the baby; we'd like to do it later as a family.

Baby Leon's Arrival

Well today is Day 8 post section and all is going well albeit a little slowly ha ha! We didn't get our VBAC unfortunately, but we did get a lot of our birth wishes and so the experience of the section wasn't too bad!

Well, I was admitted at 38+5 after pushing for more and more time from the doctors. I finally relented and also was a little worried that should my waters go Leon was at risk. So this started my 12 day hospital stay. God this was tough. My biggest concern was that I was leaving Reuben (22 months) for so long and would then return home with a new baby and I was scared this would be much more diffiuclt on him than if I had not been in hospital for so long before the birth! He visited as much as his dad could get him in and spoke to me on the phone as much as he could also, and thank goodness for my MIL who stepped in so that my DH wouldn't have to take time of before the birth!

Anyway, the events during the 10 days before the birth in the hospital were pretty uneventful! A consultant came in every morning and obs were done every couple of hours. This was so frustrating as I could still feel the baby's head under my ribs so they weren't telling me anything I didn't already know! What was very interesting though was the difference of opinion of each doctor that visited.

It was great that none were putting pressure on to make a date for a section, but some of the doctors were so condescending. I had your book with me Tracy the Guide to C sections and VBAC in Ireland and also the GentleBirth stuff. One doctor threw his eyes up to heaven when I explained what it was and another picked it up off my locker (a little rude imo) and looked disdainfully, asking me if it was any good (the same doc has written some books of his own!). And the head midwife who did the rounds was the worst. She pointed my reading material out to one of the docs who basically said to me that "a little learning is a dangerous thing". I said to him that I hoped he didn't apply the same rules to his own life given the work he does!

However I then met some other fantastic docs. I had asked about an ECV early in my stay and was told no, basically, as it wouldn't work and the baby would just turn again anyway! But on Day 6 a Dutch doc did the rounds and asked straight away if I'd considered ECV. I said I had but the docs seemed to think it would not be a good idea. He said that he was confident that there would be no issues if he were to do it, and if he could get the baby to turn he would know if the lie was stable and I could be home for Easter (the next day). So we called DH in and later that day he tried the ECV x 2. I was so excited because when he started *he said, wow the baby is turning really easily, but then scanned and was like oh no the little bugger didnt move at all! So he tried again and still no budging him. This doc then said that he really felt there was nothing else that they could do and I should schedule a section after the Bank Hol. I was a semi P patient so they wanted my own "doctor" to see me first (this never happened!). When the consultants came on Tues they decided as the ECV (or Chinese burn on the belly as one midwife described it which is kinda apt, but the hypnobirthing definitely made the experience very manageable with minimum discomfort) hadn't worked to schedule the section for the next day my due date! At this stage I was ok with it as I felt that I really had tried everything!*

So Tues (26th April) night (the night before the scheduled section) I began feeling a little funny and during the night felt like I had some pains or what felt like kinda stretching or something, but by Wed morning at about 5.00 am they were now regular and were def contractions and I lost my mucus plug too. I let the midwives know and texted DH at 5.30 am in case he needed to get in asap! I showered and prepared myself for the day and they brought me down to prep me at about 9.00 am. The contractions were now about 3-4 mins apart but there was no concern as my waters hadn't gone but the surgeon felt that we should move the surgery up a little anyway so we contacted DH and they said they would begin as soon as he got there.

Now in the week before I was hospitalised I wrote a letter to the Master expressing my birth wishes should a c section be deemed medically necessary and I had spoken to several of the lactation team around this also. My preferences were simple:

◊ *to avoid separation*

◊ *to have skin to skin as soon as possible*

◊ *to be allowed bf as soon as possible*

◊ *for the cord to be left pulsating.*

However during the 10 days prior to delivery there was very mixed attitudes to the birth wishes and I often heard that separation was likely and skin to skin was unlikely until we got back to the ward. However the lactation team were really pushing for it and were delighted to have someone so proactive about nursing as soon as possible.

So DH arrived, I was prepped, he was prepped and after the anaesthetic was put in and they were ready to begin the incision DH was brought in. The atmosphere in the theatre was calm and inclusive, everyone including the surgeons let us know what was happening at each stage and even joked a little about how stubborn babba was as they delivered his feet and could not get his little head down. The surgeon said to me at that point there was no way he could have been born any other way. When they managed to deliver Leon he was a little stunned so they had to cut the cord and use suction and oxygen and then he was happy out. Again, the whole team ensured we knew what was happening.

This is the best bit: Leon was brought over to us wrapped in the blankets we had for him and I got to kiss him. He then stayed with DH beside me which was lovely. Then before we knew it they must have finished stitching me and the atmosphere in the room became even more relaxed and lovely. I was propped up right and the baby was placed on my chest and he began to feed. The staff reduced in the room and each person that had been there congratulated us and left until there was me, DH and about two to three others, one it seemed specifically helping with latching and the others monitoring me. Essentially the OR was changed into a recovery room and there was no rushing me. Leon fed for about 45 mins and the staff took photos in the theatre, they are amazing! Then afterwards DH took Leon off to be dressed and I was brought to recovery for about 15 mins so we had our lovely family time. Leon fed and it went well and then we settled into our room.

I stayed in hospital for 48 hours after the surgery and then was let home, and since then bonding between Leon and I is going very well, BF'ing is fantastic and Reuben is delighted with his new brother! A section is not an ideal birth for so many reasons, but at least we got to have some more natural time together post birth and I feel this really helped me psychologically and emotionally. Now I need to write back to the hosp to point out all the positives and to impress upon them how great it would be if this could happen all the time for all c section mums!

VBAC: Vaginal Birth After Caesarean

The old adage "once a caesarean always a caesarean" is no longer holding true for more and more women giving birth. Worldwide VBAC (vaginal birth after caesarean) births are increasing. As women become better educated in the birthing process, more are opting for labour instead of automatically scheduling a repeat caesarean.

Is VBAC Safe?

It is possible for most women who have had a caesarean (70 to 80 per cent) to go on to have a successful vaginal birth. There is a very small risk (5 per 1,000) of uterine rupture with one low transverse scar. (most caesarean sections are performed using a cut below the bikini line; it is less disfiguring and takes less time to recover from than the previous cut from a mother's navel to her pubic bone).

Why Choose VBAC?

According to Birthrites.org: "There are many psychological effects of a caesarean birth. These continue on if the caesarean was unexpected by the mother. The loss of control, and the fear associated with an earlier birth experience, may result in the need to maintain control the next time. The amount of technology involved and the sterile atmosphere may cause a desire for a 'natural' labour and a reduction in unnecessary interventions. When women choose a VBAC birth, they tend to be making a highly informed choice."

Questions about VBAC

Q: My doctor told me my pelvis is too small to vaginally deliver a baby over eight pounds and I have to have another caesarean. Is this true?

A: No, the pelvis and the baby's head are not fixed bone structures. During labour the pelvis opens, allowing room for the baby, whose head moulds to fit. Your baby's head is made up of five quite pliable bone "plates" that overlap each other while moving through the birth canal. You've probably seen pictures of babies with cone-shaped heads. This isn't permanent; the bones will return to their prebirth state within a few hours.

The pelvis will actually open up 33 per cent larger than its pre-pregnant size with a squatting position. There are several factors that contribute to this. First a hormone called relaxin is released during the latter part of pregnancy, which softens the ligaments and cartilage surrounding the pelvis.

You may notice this during pregnancy; it can feel like arthritis in your joints. Also, different positions assumed during labour, such as walking, climbing stairs and squatting, will change the dimensions of the pelvis. This combined with the flexibility of the baby's head gives ample room for babies to move through the pelvis.

Q: I can't find a doctor willing to support a vaginal birth after caesarean.

A: Finding a doctor to be supportive can be difficult. Take the time to make an appointment and go and see several doctors. Ask questions and listen to their answers. VBACs can take a lot of work – even before labour.

Q: Doesn't a vaginal birth cause problems like pelvic floor "damage"?

A: Lead researcher Dr Alastair MacLennan in an interview with Reuters Health states: "80% of the problems a woman having a vaginal delivery has, also happen to a woman having a caesarean section." Most often it is the interventions like episiotomies, vacuum and forceps deliveries that contribute to urinary and faecal incontinence, uterine prolapse, and pelvic floor damage, rather than the vaginal birth itself. Women who have had caesarean deliveries also experience urinary and faecal incontinence and other concerns due to the surgery or simply as a result of the hormones of pregnancy and/or the drugs used during the delivery.

> Q: Wouldn't a caesarean be safer than a vaginal birth after a caesarean?
>
> A: A caesarean section is major abdominal surgery, with all that entails. The surgery itself, as opposed to medical problems that might lead to a caesarean, increases the risk of maternal death, hysterectomy, haemorrhage, infection, blood clots, damage to blood vessels, urinary bladder and other organs, postpartum depression, post-traumatic stress syndrome, and re-hospitalisation for complications.
>
> Potential chronic complications from scar tissue adhesions include pelvic pain, bowel problems, and pain during sexual intercourse. Scar tissue makes subsequent caesareans more difficult to perform, increasing the risk of injury to other organs as well as placenta previa, placenta accreta, infertility, ectopic pregnancy, uterine rupture in subsequent pregnancies and the risk of chronic problems from adhesions.
>
> There are also risks to the baby such as respiratory distress syndrome, prematurity, lower birth weights, jaundice and lower Apgar scores.
>
> *© International Caesarean Awareness Network (ICAN).*
> *Reproduced with kind permission.*

Since we know that vaginal deliveries are almost always safer for the mother, and usually as safe for the baby, and that VBAC attempts are successful in about 80 per cent of cases, why do some women still choose to have a repeat caesarean rather than try for a vaginal delivery? In some cases it is fear of pain during labour (although many patients report that the pain from recuperation from a caesarean section is worse than labour pain); in others it is a "fear of the unknown"; while for some women there is a convenience in scheduling the exact date of their baby's birth. Often a mother who has had a traumatic induction that ended in a caesarean will probably not want to repeat that experience and not even consider VBAC – without even realising that the induction itself may well have led to the caesarean.

Finally, a number of women do not wish to take the risk, no matter how rare, of uterine rupture. No matter the reason, since there is a small risk with an attempt at vaginal delivery and a risk with repeat caesarean, women should make the best choice for themselves, based on their medical history and situation.

I run the Irish ICAN (International Caesarean Awareness Network) chapter, a support group for women who have been negatively affected by caesareans. Come along to a meeting and find out how you can help yourself and others who've been through the same experience.

◇◇◇

Caelan's Birth Story

On the 6th April I visited an acupuncturist in the hope of avoiding a chemical induction in hospital and so reducing my chances of a VBAC. It was a relaxing session and I enjoyed it immensely despite being nervous to start with. The next day I had a check up and was told though changes were afoot, I would not go into labour today or tomorrow. The doctor, however agreed with my decision not to be induced until at least 14 days over so I was delighted with that and agreed I'd come back to the hospital at 9 days over for a scan and to check both my self and baby were doing well. I relaxed and myself and my husband went to a pub for some grub and I had a glass of wine, before picking up the twins from crèche. It was a lovely sunny day and we enjoyed eating outside. Interestingly, in my mind movie I had prepared for birth, I had said it was a lovely day and we ate outside before I had contractions!

Anyway, that night we went to bed and my husband gave me some of his own prostaglandin and headed off for a long sleep. I woke at 4.00 am however to the feeling of the first surge. Out comes the mobile to time them, ten mins later — another one, ten mins later another…. I got excited and told my husband who was somewhat disbelieving and put his hand on my tummy. By the time the next one came he was asleep again! By 5.30 I was too excited to sleep so I got up and watched TV and went on the internet to share my expectations with fellow April Mammies. This continued through the morning and next day and my husband went off to work. I spent the day with My sister and we went for a short walk, played with the children and I took some short naps listening to my GentleBirth tracks. After my husband came home we called my brother to stay the night and he arrived at 8.30. At this stage I was still getting surges at 10 mins apart but they seemed stronger. By 10.30 I was getting worried about the baby and why I was having surges for so long but nothing was changing. We agreed to go to the Rotunda to get checked out but if I was less than 3 cm to return home. We packed the car and headed off, stopping once to get over a strong surge.

Thankfully the hospital was a mere 15 minutes drive away so we timed the departure for just after a contraction! When we got to the Rotunda, we were sent into the emergency room and eventually checked. I was 4 cms and told I was in labour and would be brought to the delivery ward. Great! I was hooked up to a trace for 20 minutes which I found irritating as it is so much harder to deal with a surge lying down.

After a while a midwife came into me and asked me if I had discussed my birthplan with a registrar in the ante natal clinic and I said I had. She said it had a few things in it that would be outside of hospital protocol and she was surprised this hadn't been raised with me. (It had but I wasn't going to change my plan! And I had been given varied responses from each professional I had spoken to about it in the clinic anyway!) So a doctor was sent for who eventually came down and highlighted the key problem areas as refusing continuous monitoring and the time limits placed on labour. We discussed why I didn't want continuous monitoring as I didn't want my movements restricted in labour and wanted to use a shower if needed but the time limits discussion was the most fraught. She was unhappy with my calling time limits arbitrary and informed me in a not too friendly manner that they deliver x number of babies a year and their research shows that long labour leads to increased maternal and infant morbidity and mortality.

She asked me if I was willing to be in labour for 24 hours or for my child to be flat lining at birth or to have cerebral palsy? What a thing to say! Of course, I had to say, yes I am. I explained that I am not irresponsible but will not have my labour timed as long as both myself and baby were doing well and there was no indicator of distress. Anyway, eventually she covered her self with detailed patient notes which outlined what

I had been informed of and my decision and we both signed it. So off to the delivery suite, room 1, where the midwives also said that they would prefer for me to be continuously monitored but that they would agree to monitor me every 14 mins or so instead. The head midwife was supportive of my decision and said its only a 1% risk — let's not think about that. She also explained that I would feel a different pain if the scar was thinning so I ensured throughout the labour that I kept a focus on the scar and if I felt any twinge or tingling there — which thankfully I never did. At 4.00 am I was checked again and found to be still at 4 cms. I was so disappointed and then they started the talk of rupturing membranes etc and I had a frightening conversation about anaesthesia should I need it as I had been very ill after previous anaesthesia. In the end it was suggested that if I needed a section, I would have to be given an general anaesthetic. Well you can imagine the shock. We agreed that that was something I would never get over and so my notes were taken out again to write in that I had said I would prefer to have a reaction to the drugs and be sick for days afterwards than be given a general anaesthetic. At this stage I was sent to walk the halls! I was on the verge of tears, seeing my birth messed up again.

After my second walk the midwife told me not to get stressed by this but I told her that was too late, I already was. We walked again and when I came back, the head midwife came into chat to me and said she had decided I wasn't in established labour and was sending me off to the labour ward instead. This was such a relief and I was so thankful to the midwife for having the sense to see this and send me packing at 6.00 am. So off I was sent to he labour ward and given a shot of Pethadine to help me sleep. I did manage to sleep and my husband went home to come back in again at 10.00 am. That morning (Friday 9th April) I woke somewhat refreshed and relieved to be given some breathing space. When the doctors came on their rounds the consultant decided that we should have a plan and I reluctantly agreed that if nothing happened by 6.00 pm I would have my waters broken and see what happens then. At this stage I thought, I'd agree as hopefully things would be moving by then and if I wasn't happy with the decision at 6.00 pm, I could have that conversation then.

Less stress was best at this stage. About an hour later however, the registrar whom I'd met in the clinic and found very open to my discussions etc arrived into me and said that she had spoken with another consultant on duty and he had agreed that if I didn't want any intervention, there was no need to break my waters at 6.00. We'll, that was a weight off my shoulders. I thanked her and will always remember her intervention.

So, with this decision taken, it was agreed that I could move into the pre-natal ward. I was slowly moving back out of the hospital! In the pre-natal ward the pressure was totally off, I could eat as I liked and wander around freely. No body was there watching me continuously. I took another shot of Pethadine at 2.00 pm and myself and my husband slept together on the bed for about 1.5 hrs. Afterwards I had a bath and rang my mum to let her know what was happening. At 8.00 pm my husband headed off home and when he was gone I decided to take another bath. In the end I stayed there for three hours and was checked every so often as I felt that the surges were getting stronger and maybe closer together. I enjoyed these few hours by myself with nobody watching me and for each surge I poured water over my belly and used the word "relax" as a focus for my breathing, breathed in Reeee and out Laaax. My legs were tense and I shook them easily in the bath which helped release the tension. Eventually at 1 am I decided to get out of the bath as I felt I needed my TENS machine, I timed my surges and found that they were now about 3-5 minutes apart. I had the machine put on and then asked to be examined. I was 7 cms and being sent back to the delivery ward. The midwife wanted to wheel me over but I was more comfortable walking. I rang my husband to come in. I walked down to the delivery suite and the two midwives from the previous night were there and they gave me a round of applause saying 'we were wondering when you were going to come back to us!' So I was settled into room four and I rang my husband again who had fallen back asleep. I think he got a fright when I said I was in the delivery room! Another trace was put on and all was well and I got hooked up to the gas and air — I LOVE that stuff!!!! When my husband arrived I relaxed and we listened to great music they had piped into the room, I swayed to David Bowie singing "Let's Dance" and we both danced together and laughed and thought about opening a bar where entonox is piped into it. There was a lovely intimate and somewhat romantic atmosphere. The two midwives came in and out and left us to it until about 5.00 am when they decided to check and see where we were at.

The waters still hadn't broken and I was starting to breathe differently and almost feel like bearing down but not quite. When I was checked the midwife felt a lip of cervix was still there and she thought it would help if she broke my waters. At this stage I was happy for them to be broken as I wanted some of the pressure relieved and a was a little bit anxious as this was the stage where my last labour ended up in a section. Once I felt the warm swoosh of water, everything started to change and the baby's head started to descend. Before this however, I had a short while where everything stopped while we waited for something to happen. It was quite relaxing as we all sat there waiting. Once the second stage started, there was no mistaking it! The midwives encouraged me into upright positions. I started initially in the chair and then to kneeling against the back of the chair. I didn't like this position though, I found the sensations so powerful and initially I spent more time concentrating on trying to get away from them. It was like I was trying to scramble away from an animal that had suddenly been let loose inside me. This stage was like nothing I could ever have imagined. There was no pain whatsoever but the power was incredible. My husband tells me that he never heard me make the sounds I did during this stage, they were so guttural. It's interesting because throughout this stage the image of a lion kept popping into my head and between surges I would lie back and say things like Gosh, Goodness Gracious. I found the pushing tiring and I did try at times to pretend I wasn't having a surge so that I would get a break but they knew what I was up to! Even my husband mentioned it afterwards; he could se that I had been pretending not to have them!

The midwives were great at relaxing me and getting me to focus on relaxing my bottom and focusing on bearing down. I needed their coaching and my husband was great with the affirmations at this stage reminding me to release and relax and that there was a wide open space for which my baby to descend. I did put on my headphones at one stage but soon tore them off, I found them too distracting and I felt like I needed to *listen to the midwives. During one particular surge I felt what seemed like a couple of cracks internally, the midwives told me at this time that I was opening well and I knew that this was the sensation of the baby's head moving though my pelvis. At each surge my husband and the midwives reassured me and congratulated me when I opened more. I was very hot and my husband kept me cooled down with a cold flannel. My legs were very tense and the midwives massaged then between surges before placing them back on their hips for each surge. Eventually, I was told they could see the baby's head, the midwives took my hand so that I could feel his head and knowing he was this close really helped me concentrate and focus on pushing. Eventually, the head emerged and I could see the baby lying sideways. The next push and the body slithered out, what a relief. It was popped up on my chest and I checked to see if it was a boy or a girl. A little boy – our Caelan Michael had arrived.*

The third stage was managed and I found it tiring having to think about anymore pushing. The placenta was bigger than the midwives had ever seen, weighing over 1 kg. All during this time I had the baby on my chest, he was never taken from me and he had his first feed for about 20 mins before being taken to be weighed etc. He weighed 9lbs 9oz and was alert immediately. When I focussed on the music that was playing I realised it was Leonard Cohen singing "Hallelujah". How appropriate! Even though I had my own playlist, the music the hospital had piped into the room all the way through was perfect.

I had a small external tear as he came out with his hand up and this had to be sutured without anaesthesia. (I was thankful I had done my perineal massage for the last six weeks especially as I had pushed instead of breathing down.) For the first time in the whole process I felt pain and no amount of sucking on gas and air dulled that pain. I gave the poor doctor such evil looks and my husband tells me my language was quite colourful. Afterwards, I felt weak and the shower took a lot out of me. It's incredible how we can be so powerful one minute and wiped out the next. On my return I tucked into my tea and toast before being sent off to the bed which would be mine for the next three days with my son. A beautiful experience and one which so many people played a part in.

The Times They are a-Changin':
New Developments in
Maternity Care

DOMINO SCHEME

Some hospitals in Ireland now offer more flexibility in their maternity services, operating early discharge schemes, home births (also known as "domino deliveries") and midwives' clinics. These are largely pilot schemes at present. (Personally I believe pizzas and packages are delivered; babies are birthed.) You have to fulfil certain criteria to be eligible for some of the schemes.

Several maternity hospitals are currently operating a **Domino/Home Birth Scheme** in certain parts of the country. This scheme enables a few women who are deemed at "low risk of complications" to see members of a dedicated midwives' team for their antenatal visits and to have a member of this team deliver their baby, either at home or in hospital. Antenatal visits are made either to the Community Midwives' Clinic or to certain local health centres and with your GP if you are doing combined care. Additional visits are made to the woman's home. Each woman interested in the Domino/Home Birth Scheme will have a routine scan at around 18–22 weeks and a physical examination and history-taking to make sure you're suitable for the scheme. If any problems develop during the pregnancy or in labour, you will be immediately transferred back to full hosptial care (around 31 per cent of cases are transferred – the criteria for transfer are very strict). Under the Domino/Home Birth Scheme, you are entitled to an early discharge after birth, if you wish, and the midwife will visit you at home for up to a week after the birth. The scheme is free.

Early Transfer Home Scheme

This service gives new mothers the opportunity to go home within the first 36 hours following delivery – as early as six hours after the birth in some hospitals. This can be great for some women but for many first-time mums it can be terrifying. It's limited to certain areas so check with your hospital to see what is available in your area. You will be visited on a daily basis by a community midwife until your baby is five days old.

You will be released from hospital six hours following your baby's birth. The Early Transfer Home Community Midwives provide care during the antenatal period and in the days following delivery. You can opt for combined antenatal care between your obstetrician and community midwife if that suits you better.

After you have given birth you will be transferred to the postnatal ward to rest and enjoy your new addition. Let your midwives know if you would like to be discharged early. Women who go home on their first day following delivery will receive approximately four visits, while those who go home on day two will receive approximately three visits. Generally, you will be visited by the same midwife postnatally. The midwives will check you and your baby to ensure you are both well. They offer feeding advice and support, monitor baby's weight and do the heel prick test.

Another guide to maternity services in Ireland is produced by Cuidiu: The Irish Childbirth Trust. It is entitled *Consumer Guide to Maternity Services in Ireland,* and is available from Cuidiu. Cuidiu is a parent-to-parent community-based voluntary support group. These schemes are available free of charge.

Midwife-led Services

Imagine having no queues or waiting time for your antenatal appointments.

Imagine spending 30 minutes of quality time chatting about your pregnancy on the couch with your midwife.

Imagine getting to know a small group of experienced midwives and one of them is with you when you give birth.

Imagine being in labour in your own private space . . . never seeing a labour ward – just you, your partner and your midwife in a quiet comfortable suite.

Imagine having more comfort measures and pain relief options than the labour ward (epidurals are available next door to the unit if necessary).

Imagine a birth suite that is as cosy and comfy as a little apartment – but with a gigantic pool in one corner and a pull out bed for dad to stay over in the other, a fridge, kettle, ensuite bathroom, TV, beanbags and floor mats.

Imagine having 1:1 breastfeeding support in your birth suite and going home the next day with your new baby.

Imagine having home visits from your midwife providing personalized postnatal care in your home – rather than a busy postnatal ward . . .

Imagine all of this was free . . .

This is the Midwife led Unit in Drogheda & Cavan. If you're newly pregnant call the Midwife led Unit for more details.

Midwife-led care is the ideal model of care for most women having a normal pregnancy. Women who attend midwives throughout their pregnancies tend to have fewer interventions and have a lower chance of ending up with a caesarean. You'll get to know a small group of midwives throughout your pregnancy, so you'll already know the midwife who takes care of you when you have your baby. **Midwife led units (MLUs)** are supportive of active birth and have birthing pools. The rooms are set up more like a comfy hotel room than a sterile hospital, with any equipment discreetly hidden away in wardrobes. You'll be encouraged to use birth mats, exercise birth balls and, importantly, you are free to labour and birth in whatever position you want. In the unlikely event of there being a complication, there is always a consultant and paediatric team on call. You are free to go home as early as six hours after the birth and have home visits from the midwives. There are currently only two MLUs in Ireland, one in Cavan and another in Drogheda.

Doulas Do What?

A relatively new trend in Irish maternity care is the arrival of the birth **doula** or professional labour supporter. The doula's primary objective is to nurture and protect the mother's memory of her birth experience through education, physical and emotional support. The doula does not try to enforce birth plans or "advocate" for the parents – that has to come from the parents themselves – but they help parents ask the right questions. The doula empowers the parents with the knowledge to make choices that are important to them and the confidence to communicate effectively with their caregiver and the hospital staff. Doulas work with the hospital staff and can free up midwives to attend to women who need more care. While consultants, midwives and nurses have other labouring women to look after, doula support is constant throughout labour and birth, beginning in the home.

In 1989, the research team of Klaus, Kennell and Klaus did a large-scale study to investigate the use of continuous one-on-one support in labour. From the study of over 600 normal labours, they found that the use of a doula made a tremendous difference in the outcome of the birth experience. The benefits of doula support as reported by Klaus et al. included:

◊ 25 per cent shorter labours (by two hours minimum)

◊ 50 per cent fewer caesarean sections

◊ 40 per cent fewer epidurals

◊ 30 to 40 per cent decrease in the need for forceps, vacuum extraction, pitocin and narcotics.

Statistics also show that women who have positive memories of their birth are less likely to develop post-partum depression, are more positive about their babies, and are more confident in their ability to be good mothers. What a great start to your transition to motherhood!

Giving Birth at Home

Home births are on the rise, but arranging a home birth in Ireland isn't easy. We have a severe shortage of community/independent midwives and there are very few GPs who will attend a home birth. Check with your local HSE Area (formerly Health Boards) to find out what's available in your area. Where a woman chooses to have a home birth and the health board cannot provide the service, some health boards provide a home birth grant towards the cost of contracting the services of a private midwife. These days you almost need to hire your midwife before you get pregnant!

Write to your local HSE Area's Community Care Section informing them of your wish for a home birth, and requesting a list of midwives in your area. Or contact the Home Birth Association who will have all the latest and best information. Unfortunately, home birth is still not the norm in Ireland so your HSE Area may not even be as clued in as the HBA.

When you make contact with the midwife or doctor of your choice, you will need to ask them to fill out a Form of Application for Maternity Care. This will entitle you to free antenatal, delivery and postnatal services. The HSE Area will also provide you with a "maternity pack", with all you should need for a home birth.

Alternatively, you can hire a midwife privately and your antenatal, delivery and postnatal care will be provided by her. Where a woman engages the services of a private midwife for the purpose of a home birth, the HSE will contribute €2,400 towards the costs (so in some areas your home birth is free!). For a list of independent midwives, contact the Homebirth Association of Ireland. (See also the Domino scheme, as discussed on page 172.)

The Modern McBirth

by Sheila Stubbs

Hospitals are often said to be good places to give birth because of their facilities. They are well equipped and have everything a birthing couple might need readily available. But so what?

In the restaurant business, particularly the fast-food business, kitchens are designed specifically for efficient food production in order to serve the most customers with the least effort in the least amount of time. But this doesn't mean we need the same equipment to prepare meals at home! Admittedly, many of us enjoy the familiar and when we go to these restaurants we know ahead of time exactly what we will get. We also know what we will get in the hospital, since it's pretty much standard fare in all franchises. There is some variety to the menu, but you're in trouble if you find yourself in a burger place when you have your heart set on a stir-fry. Birth shouldn't have to be like a drive-thru window. "Let's see, you ordered the birthing room with a jacuzzi, and you'll need an epidural to go. You want pitocin with that?"

When you go in for your McBirth at the local franchise, you know what to expect. Nurses and doctors are there to serve you, but special orders may upset them. After all, this is their territory, and they are in charge. Because you are in their territory, you have few rights and little to do but pace the halls or lie on the assigned bed. You might be allowed to shower, but any staff member is free to walk in on you at any time.

By contrast, home birth can be like a take-out Chinese. You can sit around in your underwear or stark naked, lie down, sit, squat, dance, watch TV. Some couples prefer the quiet candlelight-and-wine atmosphere, listening to soft music while they wait until the bun is ready to come out of the oven.

Other home-birthing couples have a Birth Day Party. Just like any family celebration, there are balloons, gift-wrapped surprises for everyone, cake and champagne! The cake is prepared ahead of time, decorated and put in the freezer. The presents are bought and wrapped and waiting for the Birth Day before they can be opened, the same as we anticipate Christmas Day.

Many women find they enjoy getting ready for the baby and the celebration party afterwards to help pass the time during labour. The nice thing is, it all depends on what you want. You can call someone over to be with you to help out, or be alone; it's up to you. It's your house, and you don't have to ask permission or argue policy with anyone!

Depending on how you feel, you can spend the hours of your labour making sure the laundry is all caught up, the house is tidy, and the next meal is planned. If you don't feel up to it, of course, you don't have to do anything. But it is somehow emotionally satisfying to complete these "nesting behaviours" yourself, such as putting clean sheets on the bed, setting out the new baby's clothes, and boiling scissors to sterilize them for cutting the cord. It's exciting to get the baby's tiny clothes and nappies laid out, reminding you with each contraction that you will soon have a real, live baby wearing them!

When you birth at home, you don't have the concern about when to go to the hospital hanging over your head. Go too soon, and you'll have a long time to labour in a crowded ward, waiting for full dilation, waiting for permission to push. And without a doubt, the longer you are there, the more likely you are to have some interventions to "speed things up". Go too late and you'll have to deal with those horrendous contractions in the car; every little bump in the road is magnified so that a smooth ride seems like torture. Then you'll be asked to cooperate with admission procedures, signing papers, undressing, being examined and settled into a room when your contractions are demanding all your attention.

Believe it or not, the reason women have less need for pain relief at home birth is because of the ideas mentioned above. The midwives are the ones in an unfamiliar territory! In her own home the woman feels in control of her environment and her situation. Giving birth is perceived to be something she "does", not something that happens to her. That perception of personal power can be enough to help her handle the amazing power of contractions. Drugs? Who needs them!

Your house may not have the same set-up as the McBirth franchise, but it doesn't matter. The homemade quality and ambiance are unsurpassed.

© Reproduced with kind permission of Sheila Stubbs

HOME BIRTH CARE

Ask any mother who has had a home birth and the first thing they'll tell you is how great it is to not have to sit around hospitals for hours waiting on appointments and how they were able to get into their own bed (use their own shower) right after their baby was born. You don't have to go anywhere for antenatal visits; the midwife will come to your home – shocking, eh? Visits will last about an hour and are very easy going with lots of opportunity to get to know each other over a cup of tea, discuss birth plans and ask questions. You will get to know your midwife (midwives if in a joint/group practice) very well, and you will have the comfort of knowing she will be the one with you at the birth.

Some home birth midwives aren't comfortable with mothers giving birth in a pool. If that's important to you, then have a chat with another midwife (but be aware your choices are limited). Your partner and other children can be present and involved in the new baby's progress.

There are fewer routine high technology antenatal screenings (ultrasound scans, etc.). These can of course be arranged through a hospital if required. Your midwife is a trusted health professional available to you by telephone at all times.

Benefits of Home Birth Aftercare

◊ You or your partner and other family members will be able to stay together with your baby – in bed with a cup of tea and a packet of Hobnobs.

◊ Your other children won't be wondering where mum has disappeared to (gone to hospital).

◊ No routine procedures or arguing hospital policies – you're the boss!

◊ All your postnatal visits (baby checks and six-week checks of mother and infant) are done in the privacy of your own home.

Home Birth Midwives and Hospital Midwives: What's the Difference?

Midwifery is a profession, totally independent of nursing (although in Ireland it used to be the case that anybody who wanted to become a midwife would have to complete training as a nurse first). Practising independent midwives are able to take sole responsibility for the care of mainly healthy women and babies, whereas nurses care for sick people, usually under the direction of doctors. (Remember, you are pregnant, not ill.) Your midwife is the specialist in normal maternity care. I know I keep repeating this, but it's important: most women (80 per cent or more) have problem-free pregnancies and labours. Your midwife is trained to be able to recognise possible problems early on. If a problem does come up, your midwife will arrange a transfer to the hospital. Hospital midwives don't get to see a lot of normal births; they do see lots of inductions, epidurals and episiotomies – so no wonder some of them see birth as a medical condition. If that was all you are exposed to, then that's your reality.

Is Home Birth Safe?

Yes. Home birth is a prime example of how our actions are affected (or not) by factual realities (scientific data) or perceptual reality (beliefs). When someone mentions home birth, do you automatically think to yourself, "How irresponsible – what if something goes wrong?" or do you think, "Excellent, this woman knows her stuff?" For the majority it's probably the former. Many people ask if home birth is safe. Our society views labour and birth as an illness or medical condition that needs to be fixed or cured. Since the beginning of time, we have given birth without medical help or intervention.

The World Health Organisation (WHO) says:

> It has never been scientifically proven that the hospital is a safer place than home for a woman who has had an uncomplicated pregnancy to have her baby. Studies of planned home births in developed countries with women who have had uncomplicated pregnancies have shown

sickness and death rates for mother and baby equal to or better than hospital birth statistics for women with uncomplicated pregnancies.

So are you perfectly safe delivering at home? Carl Jones (author of *Childbirth Choices Today*) states:

> There is always going to be some risk when giving birth, as in all of life, and women should be carefully screened for any health problems that could be dangerous during labour and delivery. For certain women in rare circumstances, obstetric care is essential. However, for most women, better, healthier results are seen when mothers choose to birth at home.

If you are a woman with no health problems or contraindications to safe labour and delivery, consider birthing at home.

Need an Extra $25,000?

Jock Doubleday, a birth activist from the US, made this offer recently:

I, Jock Doubleday, will pay $25,000.00 (US) to the first person who sends me, both by email and postal mail, a study published in an industry journal in any country, in any time period, demonstrating hospital birth to be safer, in any category (i.e., infant or maternal mortality or morbidity), for most mothers and babies than home birth with a trained midwife in attendance. The term "midwife" does not include Certified Nurse Midwives, who, because of their conventional medical training, and in spite of their good intentions, may bring the fear-based medical model of childbirth with them into the home, thus skewing home birth data toward the technological. Fear, in any guise, is contagious. This offer has no expiration date and supersedes all previous offers of a similar nature. Contact: jockdoubleday@aol.com.

So why is there still an assumption that hospital is safer than home? The fact is, supporters of active management of labour point to the fact that, in the past, where fewer interventions were available, mortality rates for mothers and newborns were much higher. But this is really accounted for by improvements in living standards, nutrition, general health and antenatal care; and these factors apply equally as well to hospital as home births.

In the UK the perinatal mortality rate for home birth compares very favourably with that of births in general:

◊ Home births: 4-5 in 1000

◊ Hospital births: 9-10 in 1000.

The following quote is from the *UK Health Committee Second Report House of Commons: Maternity Services, Vol. 1 (The Winterton Report)*, published in March 1992:

> On the basis of what we have heard, the committee must draw the conclusion that the policy of encouraging all women to give birth in hospital cannot be justified on grounds of safety.

The *British Medical Journal* of 23 November 1996 published a Swiss study, "Home vs. Hospital deliveries: follow up study of matched pairs for procedures and outcome". Their key conclusions include:

> There are no obvious disadvantages of home delivery for mother or child when the mother opts for home delivery.

A landmark study released in 2005 again backed up all the positive recommendations about home birth and safety ("Outcomes of planned home births with certified professional midwives: large prospective study in North America", Kenneth C. Johnson, senior epidemiologist, Betty-Anne Daviss, project manager, *BMJ*, 2005, 330:1416 (18 June), doi:10.1136/bmj.330.7505.1416.

In some areas of Ireland, mothers-to-be have to make round trips of 100 miles to attend antenatal clinics in hospital. This is due to closures of smaller maternity units and the running down of domiciliary services.

Apart from the obvious inconvenience of travelling such distances, there are other risks involved – long and high-speed car journeys to hospital; giving birth unattended either at home or on the roadside, which is particularly applicable on second or subsequent babies, where labours can be very short and fast.

Given these risks, some women choose induction in order to avoid either of these scenarios. Inductions themselves come with risks, so it becomes a Catch-22 situation: take the "risk" of having a home birth, which has been proven safe for most women; or make your life miserable by racing to a hospital mid-labour; or opt for an unnecessary early induction that might not work! In these cases, it makes sense to have your baby at home with a local midwife (provided you can find one).

Benefits of Having a Home Birth:

◊ You're in your own home; it doesn't get any better than that!

◊ If you have other children they can be at the birth, as can your partner, sister, best friend or even great-granny!

◊ Nobody will be watching the clock or trying to rush your labour.

◊ You have your baby your way; no wondering if you are "allowed" to birth on the floor or swinging from the chandeliers if that's what floats your boat.

◊ You can labour in a birth pool.

◊ No routine procedures.

◊ You'll be more relaxed (less adrenaline) so your body will labour more effectively.

All of these benefits also reduce complications in childbirth for you and your baby: less foetal distress diagnoses; fewer babies needing resuscitation; fewer low Apgar scores at one minute (a check on the baby's well-being); less incidence of post-partum haemorrhage in the mother.

<<<<<<<<<<<<<<<<<<<<<<<<<<<<<<<<<<<<<<<<<<<<<<<<<<<<<<<<<<<<<<<<<<<<<<<<<<<<<<<<<<<<<<<<<<

Maria's Birth Story

I was eight days overdue for the birth of my second child. We had planned a home birth in my mom's house, as this put us in the catchment area for the Community Midwives from the National Maternity Hospital. This was to be my partner's first birth experience and our six-year-old daughter was very excited and prepared.

I had spent the last two days with mild contractions during the day, getting stronger towards the evening, but then stopping throughout the night – quite frustrating. I had been leaking a bit of amniotic fluid, but the midwives had said the forewaters were intact and that perhaps it was a small leak from the hindwaters but that I could still wait until things kick-started. I had recently been stuck in traffic for two hours, so we decided to stay over in mom's, just in case.

On the Friday I woke up at 5.30 am, having had the best night's sleep in ages. I left Paul and Ella to sleep. Contractions started coming every five to six minutes, about 45 seconds long and more significant than the ones the previous days, so I rocked on the birth ball in the living room.

At about 6.00 am Paul woke up and joined me, He rubbed my back as I rocked. My mom woke up at about 7.00, and moved a still sleeping Ellie from the bed we were planning to use, which was a double-bed mattress on the floor in the dining room. Paul called the midwives who said that the new shift midwife would be there shortly and that she would call back when she arrived.

She did call at 7.30 and said that she and her second midwife were going to leave for us straight away. I was in the bath while Paul talked to them, and mom poured water across my tummy. The contractions were coming hot and heavy and I started to find the bath too restrictive and was unable to kneel on all fours, my more comfortable position. I went back downstairs and knelt on the mattress on the floor, leaning over the birth ball. Ella had woken by now and came in to give me a kiss. She asked if I was OK and I said, yes, baby will be here soon, and she said that she and Grandma were going to go make the baby a birthday cake and card.

At 8.15 the midwife called again, asking if everything was OK, and letting us know she was ten minutes away. Paul was rubbing my back and reassuring me, "They'll be here soon" – between bouts of muttering, "Where the *#$* are they?"

At about 8.30 the contractions changed, I felt the overwhelming urge to push, I pushed away the birth ball. I needed solid ground. "Stop," I told Paul who was rubbing my back. I felt I needed to make sure that it was time to push without any other stimulus. "That was different; I have to push."

I had been hoping that the midwives would get there in time but now I knew that we were on our own. I felt a panic, for Paul; how would he cope with this? Then I had to settle down to do the job. My waters broke, I heard Paul call my mom for towels. As mom walked into the room with the towels, I heard Paul exclaim, "I can see the head!" It seemed like only a couple more pushes until Paul said, "The head's out, what do I do?"

"Is there a cord?" I asked. He said he could see one. Two more pushes and out came baby, caught by Paul's able hands.

I was still on all fours. Paul told me to lie down but I couldn't, I was too wobbly. He had to tip me over onto my side, then he handed me the baby and threw a blanket over us, and lay down beside me. We lay there quietly looking at the baby, who had opened its eyes and whimpered a bit.

Mom and Ella came in. Ella cleaned a small patch on the baby's head and kissed it, then lay down beside us. We then realised that we didn't know what sex the baby was. It was a girl; I had been sure that it was go-ing to be a boy but Paul and Ella had chosen a girl's name, Abby Anna.

The midwife arrived ten minutes later, 9.00. My mom met them at the door saying, "She's here," to which the midwife replied, "Oh yes, I'm sorry were late." Mom said, "No, the baby – she's here!"

The midwives came in and sat watching us for another ten minutes before they did anything, just chatting, helping to get baby latched on, and looking, taking in the information. I was happy they didn't come in and "take over". They then cut the cord, but I would have wanted them to of-fer it to Paul to do, a last final job to do. Then they checked and weighed Abby, 8 lbs, 11 oz, and helped Patrick to dress her and also helped me to birth the placenta and checked the perineum for any damage, helped me clean up, have a shower, etc.

I spent the rest of that day in bed. I felt great and my family kept saying how great I looked. It was so nice to have Ella there too. Next time she wants to be in the room for the birth. Paul, at this time, had lost his knees, he kept saying, "But what if something had gone wrong?" It took him a long time to get over that shock. Even now, he doesn't like to think about what might have been. He has agreed to go for a home birth again next time – but this time with the midwife!

I felt and still feel completely empowered by this experience; this is what my body is made to do and I did it without any medical involvement. I often wonder how many other births become medicalised when, if left to instinct they would have turned out as well as my experience. I'm dying to do it all again; I'm afraid I could get addicted to being pregnant, giving birth and having children!

Lotus Birth

By Sarah Buckley

Lotus birth is the practice of leaving the umbilical cord uncut, so that the baby remains attached to his/her placenta until the cord naturally separates at the umbilicus – exactly as a cut cord does – at three to ten days after birth. This prolonged contact can be seen as a time of transition, allowing the baby to slowly and gently let go of his/her attachment to the mother's body.

Although we have no written records of cultures that leave the cord uncut, many cultures hold the placenta in high esteem. For example, Maori people from New Zealand bury the placenta ritually on the ancestral marae, and the Hmong, a hill tribe from South East Asia, believe that the placenta must be retrieved after death to ensure physical integrity in the next life: a Hmong baby's placenta is buried inside the house of its birth.

Things to consider if you're planning a Lotus birth.

◊ "Ugggggh ..." is a typical response, and you'll get sick of hearing it very quickly! It might be easier to not tell anyone. Many couples who plan lotus birth see the days with the placenta (usually four to six days) as private family time and make a rule that they will not have guests until the placenta is separated. This relieves the new mother of performance anxiety as she gets to know her new baby. It gives the baby a quiet transition period to intensively bond with his/her parents. One couple I know did not let anyone know their baby had been born until the placenta had separated naturally.

◊ What if it smells terrible? Ground rosemary sprinkled all over the surfaces gives the placenta a pleasant smell like turkey stuffing. (Hope you're feeling festive!) There will be a smell. It is not terrible. A cake rack can be helpful to place the placenta on to allow air to circulate. Nappies are helpful to prevent bedclothes from being stained with blood. The placenta is organ meat that is fresher than any meat you have ever purchased. It will naturally begin to smell after a few days of being in the air. Sometimes keeping it in a casserole dish in cold water can help too.

◊ What if I decide not to do it once I've started? Not a problem. The cord can be cut at any time and usually is atrophied (dried and shrunk) enough that it needs no clamp after 24 hours. It is common for new parents to go through periods where they think Lotus birth is just too much trouble. Often the mother wants to give up and cut the cord and the father will talk her into persisting a while longer; then, the father can be fed up and the mother will encourage him to keep going. It becomes a quiet meditation to wait vigilantly for the cord to fall and in our fast-moving society it is a real contest to slow down for the baby. Parents report that the days spent with the placenta attached taught them a great deal about cooperative parenting and patience.

◊ What are the annoying aspects of Lotus birth? It can seem like a nuisance to have to move the placenta every time you move the baby. Having a piece of raw meat in your family bed is a little peculiar, too, and can be messy. Once the cord dries after 24 hours, it has the consistency of rawhide, which makes it seem like your baby has a wire coat hanger protruding from his/her belly. None of these problems is insurmountable if the parents can be relaxed, stay close to bed and view Lotus Birth as a rite of passage.

> ◊ How do I do this with a three-year-old jumping around on the bed? This is actually one of the biggest challenges and is a reason that Lotus birth most often happens with first births. Protecting the newborn from the exuberance of a three-year-old is not easy at the best of times. Prior to the birth, the parents should put some thought into creating a "nest" for the new baby and mom for the Lotus time. The father and older child can build a "play space" of some kind with new library books and music for nap times. Enlisting friends and family to take the older child for some active outdoor fun each day will also help the new parents maintain the sanctity of the Lotus time for the baby.
>
> © *Reproduced with kind permission of Sarah Buckley and Birthlove.com*

WATER BIRTH

In the same way that a nice soak in a warm bath can melt away muscle tension and the stress of the day, using warm water in labour has a wonderful effect and allows for a more gentle entry into the world for your baby. Michel Odent pioneered the birth pool in France in the early 1960s and the use of birthing pools has grown steadily ever since. Using water during labour helps relax you so labour can progress normally. It takes the weight off your limbs so you can change positions very easily and the water makes you feel much lighter (can't be a bad thing when you've been pregnant for nine or even ten months). If you're planning a home birth then getting a pool these days is very easy. Birth pools come in all shapes and sizes – the deeper the better.

Take a wander through your house to decide where to put your birth pool. Most mums like to labour in an enclosed area that is not too big – so right in the middle of the living room might not feel like the best place during labour. If you're birthing upstairs, then make sure your floor can take the weight of the water! You will probably also want to avoid any rooms with brand new white or light-coloured carpet. The room should be big enough so that your midwife can have easy access if needs be.

Depending on your heating system, you may need to keep the immersion on permanently so you can be sure the pool is warm enough. Ideally, the water should be maintained around 37 degrees Celsius and no higher; otherwise you're likely to overheat and it can affect the baby.

If you don't have a birth pool, your bathtub will do but it's not ideal. You'll want to be sure that you have someone with you to help you in and out, and a non-slip mat. The tub is a bit of a tight squeeze if your partner or other children wanted to join you.

In Russia you can even hire transparent acrylic pools. The video Birth into Being follows several midwives who host a "birth camp" at the edge of the Black Sea each summer; the babies are born into the warm ocean. I can't see many Irish mothers blazing a trail to Dollymount to give birth!

The recommended rental period is for four weeks – two weeks before and after estimated date of arrival. The cost is approximately €120. If using a pool with a disposable liner, you buy this for around €40. It is now also possible to purchase one-time use pools for €57. Delivery can be arranged for about €43. Check on e-Bay too; you might get a bargain.

Talk to your midwife about your plans to use a birth pool. Find out if she has had previous experience and how she feels about birthing in the water as opposed to only labouring in water (if this is your choice). If you are planning to use a pool don't focus completely on giving birth in the water. Some mothers like to get out of the water and birth "on dry land". You won't know how you will feel until you get to that stage but don't make it a project just so you can have a water birth. As with the rest of labour, if it feels right then listen to what your body is telling you.

Tips for Getting Ready

Put a plastic tarp under the pool. You can also use a flannel-backed vinyl tablecloth (flannel side up) under the pool, especially the side you will be getting in/out of most, to stop you slipping. Throw down a few sheets or towels on top of the tarp. Give your local St Vincent de Paul a call and get some old sheets/towels from them. You'll just be throwing them out anyway, so you won't want to use your good linen!

When using an inflatable pool, put the cold water in first – then the hot water. Get a thermometer (buy one that you can use for your newborn's bathtime) to test the temperature. Always fill it a quarter of the way with room temperature water, then add your hot water. You need to keep the temperature around 37 degrees celsius. This will keep the plastic in the tub from melting (a high priority!) and enable you to monitor the temperature of the water better. Keep an eye on the temperature coming out of the hose, too, to make sure your water heater isn't out of hot water!

It's vital to stay well hydrated and get out of the pool if you get dizzy or lightheaded. Keep a few ice cold washcloths by the pool and in the fridge. Have a few fruit juice and water ice pops already made in the freezer (you probably won't be in the mood for a Wibbly Wobbly Wonder). Keep a bowl of ice with just a bit of water that you can put a couple of washcloths in – your body temperature will warm up those cloths quickly, so get your partner to change them often!

It's better to avoid putting any aromatherapy oils in the pool. An option is to have a mister (spray bottle) with some cool, distilled water and a few drops of essential oil instead. It's much easier to get rid of a spray bottle than to have the entire house smelling of lavender from the steam of the tub and in the birth tub itself. And it can make you sick, as your sense of smell is heightened during labour.

© *Pamela Hines-Powell and Circle of Life Midwifery,*
www.midwifemama.com. Reproduced with kind permission.

What is the Baby's Experience of Being Born in Water?

Being born in water makes birth a very gentle process for your baby. He will not take his first breath until he reaches the surface, so there's no need to worry about your baby drowning. As far as he's concerned, he's still just floating in amniotic fluid – except that the womb just got a whole lot bigger! Birthing in the pool makes it easier to catch your own baby too (often with the guidance of your midwife). Research has shown that being born in water is a safe alternative for low-risk mothers with no medical issues (as long as mum and baby are doing well).

The Third Stage of Labour

The first few hours after birth is a critical time for you and your baby to get to know each other. Coincidentally, it's within the first hour of birth that your baby is most alert and this is the best time to start breastfeeding. What you and your baby need most from each other at this time is eye contact, skin-to-skin contact and lots of cuddles. This is a brand new world to your baby so he has a lot to get used to very quickly but you can make the transition easier by keeping your baby with you. Many hospitals now see the benefits of "rooming-in" instead of automatically sending your baby to the nursery unless there is a medical need. If your baby has to go to the nursery, have your partner go with him. Co-sleeping is not encouraged in hospitals especially if the mum has had a tiring labour and is taking medication. Co-sleeping is fantastic for breastfeeding once you get home, as it means you'll get more sleep and feel better rested during the day. It's sometimes referred to as "dreamfeeding".

THE THIRD STAGE: DELIVERING THE PLACENTA

The **third stage of labour** refers to the part of labour and delivery most people forget – the birth of the placenta. As with most areas of labour, you have the choice of delivering the placenta naturally or having an actively managed third stage.

An actively managed third stage involves an injection of syntocinon into the mother's thigh. A natural third stage occurs when no drugs are administered and the baby's suckling results in the release of oxytocin, which causes the uterus to contract. As long as the placenta separates from the uterine wall, there is no rush to deliver it, as once it has peeled away from the wall of the uterus, there is a lower risk of haemorrhage. A doctor or midwife can easily tell whether or not the placenta has separated by gently palpating the fundus (top of the uterus). If the cord does not move, then the placenta has indeed separated from the uterine wall.

There is no need to cut the cord until the placenta has been delivered, unless it is not long enough to allow the baby to suckle, or it has become wrapped around the baby's neck in several loops. In the latter case, most of the time the cord can just be unlooped (it's quite common for a baby to be born with the cord around his neck and is easily fixed). In most instances, the placenta will be delivered shortly after birth.

CARE OF THE CORD

The umbilical cord carries blood from the placenta to the newborn, and continues to do so until the cord has stopped pulsating. It is therefore not a good idea to cut the cord before it has stopped pulsating. The cord will usually stop pulsating in about five minutes. Policy in most Irish hospitals is to cut the cord immediately.

Once the cord has been successfully cut and clamped, there is no need to give it any special care. Cord spirit, for example, is entirely unnecessary and can even irritate the baby's skin. If anything, just apply a few drops of breastmilk to the site – this will stave off infection and will be kind to your baby's skin.

CORD STEM CELL COLLECTION

Another new option in Ireland for parents is cord stem cell collection. If you decide to preserve your baby's stem cells then you need to also look at the risks to him of early cord cutting which reduces your baby's blood volume significantly.

Stem Cells: What Are They Used For?

Stem cells have proven their use in the treatment of a growing number of serious, life-threatening diseases. Until recently, in the case of malignant blood disorders such as leukaemia, doctors could only hope for a bone marrow transplant in order to boost the number of healthy blood cells in the patient. However, bone marrow transplants are not always possible. The injection of stem cells has been shown to be a valid alternative to bone marrow transplants, especially in children and adolescents.

The advantage of preserving cord blood stem cells is: (a) their immediate availability, even years later; (b) there is no risk of rejection, as the healing cells are one's own; and (c) the whole process is entirely safe and drug-free. As such, it builds on a natural process.

At the moment it is believed that stem cells will play a major role in various medical fields. Stem cells lead to the renewal of several types of tissues: blood, muscle, nerve and liver cells, bone and cartilage tissues. Stem cells could be applied directly to the damaged tissue at the exact site of the damage, without drugs. For example, following a heart attack, transplanting stem cells directly at the site of the infarction has been noted to offer benefit to the outcome of the disease.

There are also strong indications but not proof yet that stem cells will be able to tackle diseases like Parkinson's, Alzheimer's, multiple sclerosis and diabetes. These diseases essentially occur when a cell type is missing, or has stopped being produced, and the stem cells "step in" to replace them. The results of stem cell treatment seem permanent. Gene therapies could correct some hereditary diseases, but can only be performed with one's own stem cells.

Keeping in mind the direction both medicine and stem cells are going, preserving your child's stem cells merits consideration; but early cord cutting reduces the blood volume to your baby by up to a third and can increase the risk of anaemia – something to consider.

© Medicare Rental and Sales, www.medicare.ie

The actual collection of the blood isn't difficult but it will affect your decisions about whether to go with a natural third stage (no medical intervention) or a managed third stage and have the syntocinon injection. When you have a managed third stage your baby's cord must be clamped immediately. Your consultant will collect the cord blood from the umbilical cord and it doesn't cause any pain to you or your baby. All in all, the procedure takes a few minutes and you can be cuddling your newborn while it's going on. The blood is then labelled and couriered to the UK, as there are no facilities in Ireland to store the stem cells. Be sure to check with your consultant and hospital if they support this procedure; some hospitals don't. The cost is approx €1,400.

Newborn Tests and Screening

If the baby is born in an Irish hospital, it is usual to carry out screening for metabolic disorders (the Guthrie or heel prick test). If the baby is born at home, the test may be carried out by the GP or in the out-patients department of a hospital.

Heel Prick Test

This is a routine screening test for all newborn babies which screens your baby for various metabolic conditions including **PKU** and more recently Cystic Fibrosis. Several drops of blood are taken from your baby's heel and dropped onto a special card that is sent to Temple Street Hospital. Before the test is done warm your baby's foot up with two pairs of socks and gently massage your baby's leg in a downward motion to make the procedure as quick as possible. Hold your baby close to you and offer the breast to comfort and re-assure your baby (breastmilk has pain-relieving properties) while the midwife does the test. Some staff offer to take your baby away to the nursery to do this test as it can be stressful on you (and staff!) – but it's also stressful on your new baby so go with your baby.

Vaccinations

Most vaccinations are not given until your baby is at least two months old. However, if your baby is at risk of tuberculosis (TB) you may be offered the option of a BCG shot shortly after birth. Vaccinations given at two months, and again at four and six months, reduce the risk of diphtheria, whooping cough, Hib, tetanus and polio. Vaccinations against measles, mumps and rubella (German measles) are usually given when your baby is about a year old. If you have concerns about possible side effects of vaccinations, discuss these with you doctor. However, it is important to stress that the risks of not vaccinating often outweigh the risks of your baby developing any side effects.

VITAMIN K

Vitamin K is routinely given in Irish hospitals. Vitamin K is mostly given so that your baby's blood will clot, and it also helps protect against a fatal disease known as newborn haemorrhagic disease, which occurs about 4–7 times per 100,000 births. Your baby will be given an intramuscular shot (usually in the thigh) of vitamin K as a precaution. Some experts feel that vitamin K is a way to ensure that any baby with haemorrhagic disease will be safe. A Japanese study showed that babies who consume 350 ml of breastmilk in the first three days following birth are protected against vitamin K deficiency. There is some dispute about the wisdom of giving high levels of vitamin K to a newborn baby, and there are also possible risks associated with the carrier substance, which has not been fully researched. Vitamin K is also available orally.

CIRCUMCISION

Circumcision of baby boys is not routinely done in Ireland, nor has it been part of our culture to circumcise babies. With the increased number of immigrants into the country and the resulting number of cross-cultural unions, it is becoming a subject that more and more Irish people are giving thought to.

Contrary to common belief, circumcision is not dictated by any religion. In some, such as Islam and Judaism, it is recommended but not mandatory.

The fact is that to circumcise the penis of a young boy is to subject him to an unnecessary operation that is, at best, extremely uncomfortable for days afterwards and, at worst, fatal. To amputate a boy's foreskin is to mutilate his genitals and serves no medical or hygienic purpose. Contrary to popular lore, a circumcised penis is not more sensitive than an uncircumcised one. The glans, which is exposed after circumcision, is not actually skin and must toughen up and desensitise after this operation. In fact, the foreskin is intended to protect this sensitive tip of the penis and to remove it does nobody any favours.

Breast is Not "Best" – It's Just Normal

If you're planning to breastfeed, it's a great idea to start learning about it before your little one arrives. There are some things you need to know that will help make breastfeeding a great experience right from the start, so let's start with some boobology. You may have gone to antenatal classes or read a few books about breastfeeding, but just like driving, reading about it or watching someone else do it isn't quite the same as doing it yourself.

As Janet Tamaro says in her book So *That's What They're For*, choosing between breastmilk and formula is like asking, "Would you rather have perfectly created, safe, chemical-free organic nutritious food or IV fluid?" We can't make blood, hearts, kidneys, livers, eyes or anything else that humans need in a factory. Only human beings make the perfect parts. And only human beings make the perfect food for their babies. Think about it – how would the human race have survived for the last million years before bottles were invented?

WHAT'S SO SPECIAL ABOUT BREASTMILK?

The current level of breastfeeding in Ireland is still around 40 per cent; a rate which is very low in comparison to rates of 99 per cent in Norway, 96 per cent in Germany and 71 per cent in the United Kingdom. However, a Lansdowne Market Research survey into breastfeeding patterns and attitudes in Ireland in 2003 revealed that 63 per cent of Irish mothers and mothers-to-be feel that breastfeeding is better than formula feeding. It is now government policy to promote breastfeeding, and a number of initiatives have been introduced, such as "Babies Who Lunch" – welcoming and facilitating breastfeeding mothers in restaurants and hotels.

We think of formula as a good second choice. But it's not even a good third or fourth choice. Yet we are led to believe that breastmilk and formula are almost equal. You don't have to love the idea of using your breasts as your child's first refrigerator, or commit to breastfeeding your little one until he's making his first communion. Before you make up your mind not to do it, make sure it's an educated decision.

You've probably heard something along the lines of, "What's wrong with formula? I was formula fed and I turned out OK!" Fair enough, but you'd be more "OK" if you'd been breastfed. Years ago, it was quite acceptable for children to bounce around the back seat of the car (and sometimes the front) with no car seats, or even seatbelts, either – and most of us did OK. But we know better now.

Studies have shown unequivocally that breastfeeding decreases the incidence of the following:

◊ Gastrointestinal and urinary tract infections

◊ Lower respiratory tract illnesses

◊ Otitis media (ear infections)

◊ Bacterernia and meningitis.

Breastfeeding has also been shown to lower infant mortality and reduce the frequency of certain chronic diseases later in life (i.e. insulin dependent diabetes, Crohn's disease, ulcerative colitis and certain lymphomas). Among the benefits occurring to a mother who breastfeeds for four to six months are a lower risk of both breast and uterine cancer.

As Breastfeeding.org states, "breastfeeding provides ideal nutrition, growth hormones and infection-fighting factors which change over time as the growing infant and child's needs change; provides it inexpensively, and with no harm to the environment. Breastfed infants are healthier overall, and research is indicating that the health benefits may continue into adulthood." Virtually every woman will be able to breastfeed her infant – even those with inverted nipples and those who have had breast augmentation or reduction surgery. If breastfeeding is difficult or painful, don't give up – get help. There's lots of support out there.

Some Truths about Breastmilk

◊ Breastmilk is always available, does not need mixing or sterilising and is always at the right temperature.

◊ Breastmilk meets all of your child's nutritional needs.

◊ Breastmilk will not be recalled by the manufacturer, has no "best before" date and will not harm your baby.

◊ Breastmilk will be a familiar taste to your baby, as it tastes like amniotic fluid, so the baby will be born liking it.

◊ There is no waste when you breastfeed your baby.

◊ Breastmilk reduces the likelihood of your child becoming obese.

◊ Breastmilk has more than 100 (some sources say more than 400) ingredients not found in formula, including at least four unique proteins. There are unique and powerful immune-building properties in breastmilk, and it can enhance brain development.

◊ Breastmilk is a living substance. Each woman's milk is individually tailored for her own baby. What's more, her milk changes constantly — both during a feed and day-by-day — to meet her baby's evolving needs. When a mother is exposed to pathogens in the environment, she produces antibodies to combat them. The mother's antibodies are then passed on to her baby via her breastmilk. (*Source*: World Alliance for Breastfeeding Action: "Breastfeeding; World Breastfeeding Week, 1997 — Nature's Way")

◊ Breastmilk is easier to digest than any alternative, which means less spitting up, vomiting, painful gas and colic.

◊ Breastmilk is the most ecological food available to humans. There is less consumption of natural resources and landfill space. The production of packaging of formula uses paper, glass, plastic and metals, all of which need to be produced and disposed of. Then there is the plastic and silicone involved in the production of the bottles and teats — not to mention the phosphates used, or water wasted, in sterilising all the equipment.

◊ Breastmilk can successfully be used to treat eye infections.

◊ Breastmilk is the only fluid that is not harmful if it gets into the lungs.

◊ Breastfeeding encourages correct growth and development of oral muscles, facial bones and promotes healthier teeth.

◊ Breastfeeding boosts women's self-reliance and self-esteem; by meeting the needs of their infants, they increase their confidence in their ability to parent and nurture.

◊ Breastfeeding protects against SIDS (cot death).

◊ Breastfed babies have up to 50 per cent fewer ear infections than bottle-fed babies

◊ Breastfeeding stimulates a mother's body to produce prolactin and oxytocin, the "mothering hormones". (Prolactin helps you feel relaxed, loving and calm. Prolactin levels can increase 10–20 fold within 30 minutes of beginning a nursing session.)

◊ The skin-to-skin contact offered by breastfeeding reduces the stress which babies experience when they enter the world from the warmth and safety of the womb.

◊ Breastfeeding enhances vaccine effectiveness.

◊ Breastfeeding reduces parental leave from work, as the baby is usually healthier.

◊ Breastfed girls have a reduced chance of suffering breast cancer in adulthood.

◊ Breastfeeding increases your oxytocin levels which help your uterus to contract to expel the placenta after birth.

© www.parentingweb.com. Adapted and reproduced with kind permission.

TIPS FOR SUCCESS

Get your baby to the breast as soon as possible – immediately if you can. Even though it doesn't seem much, **colostrum** is all your baby needs for the first few days, until your milk "comes in"; he's not thirsty and he's not very hungry. (You may have noticed that your breasts leaked a little in the last few weeks before birth: this is colostrum. This "liquid gold" is highly concentrated with nutrients and antibodies to nourish and protect your newborn).

Newborns are usually alert for about an hour after birth (some babies may be drowsy from the epidural, if you have had one). Take advantage of this time, as your baby will be very interested in your breast. Put it in your birth plan that this is very important to you. Make sure your baby isn't routinely taken away for observation, unless there is a real medical need. Try to keep your baby with you; being separated from you is upsetting. After all, he's been with you his whole life. He's just moved house and we all know how stressful that can be; your baby is just getting used to his new surroundings. Don't let friends or relatives talk you into sending your baby off to the nursery so you can get some rest. As tired as you are, your baby needs you. If you need help with the latch (attaching your baby to the breast properly so that it doesn't hurt), ask to see the hospital lactation consultant or your midwife. When you get home, contact the La Leche League for help or a private lactation consultant. Not all public health nurses have the experience needed to help a new mum with a breastfeeding problem.

I remember watching an amazing documentary from Sweden in which a newborn baby, less than an hour old, actually crawls to the nipple of his mother with no assistance at all – sensing her breastmilk by smell.

Within a few days of giving birth, you may well wake up in the middle of the night with two hot bowling balls instead of breasts (hot being the temperature, and it's bloody uncomfortable). This often happens when your milk comes in initially. The great news is that it's easy to fix and only temporary. An easy way to help with engorgement is first of all for Dad to take the baby and you take a warm shower or get a nice warm moist towel and gently massage your breasts and the milk will begin to flow. Then, as soon as you can, get baby on the breast for his first big meal.

Don't be alarmed if your baby seems to be constantly on the breast for the first three or four days. This does not mean the baby isn't getting enough – on the contrary, it means that the baby is so well satisfied with what you are producing for her that she can't stay away! Hungry babies cry – if your baby is constantly suckling but does not seem to be upset or distressed, then she is not hungry.

How Do I Know if She is Getting Enough Milk?

Wouldn't it be so much easier if our babies came with a fluid indicator, like the petrol gauge in your car? Well it's actually simple physics – you can measure your baby's input by his output! Your baby may have only one or two wet nappies during the first day or two after birth. On about the third or fourth day, she will have at least five or six really wet nappies (six to eight if you're using cloth). A week later, 8–12 wet nappies is the norm.

The Scoop on Poop

Meconium, the greenish-black, tarry first stool, will be passed by the baby in the first day or two. (Colostrum is a natural laxative, and will help with the passing of this first stool.) Your baby will begin to have between three and five bowel movements a day, starting on or about the third day after birth. Breastfed babies tend to have yellow mustardy poops that don't smell, because breastmilk is easily digested. Breastfed babies are more "regular" than formula-fed babies. For the first year of his life, my son pooped to a schedule; we could almost time it.

During the first few days after birth, your baby may lose up to ten per cent of her birth weight. Some of this is "water weight" caused by the extra fluids taken by Mum with an epidural so your baby's weight may have been slightly inflated to begin with. Once your milk supply becomes more plentiful on the third or fourth day, she will start to gain. Generally, babies gain 170g (6oz) per week. Be sure to count weight gain from the lowest weight (i.e. the baby's weight on the third or fourth day), not from birth weight.

The best way of knowing if your baby is getting enough is that she will be obviously healthy, her skin will be firm and of a healthy colour, she will be filling out and growing in length and head circumference. She will be alert and active.

If you experience any pain or discomfort when breastfeeding, or have any worries about your supply, seek help immediately. Your local branch of La Leche League is an excellent form of support and you may even be lucky to find a lactation consultant either through a maternity hospital or independently.

Look at the Baby Not the Scale

In the first 24 to 72 hours after birth babies tend to lose about 3-10% of their birth weight and then regain that weight over the next 2 to 3 weeks. If a mother receives lots of IV fluids during labour, the baby could be born "heavier" because of the increased water. The somewhat higher weight could be measured if a baby were weighed right before it peed for the first time. The difference of this extra fluid retention might only be a few ounces, but some parents are told to be concerned when, at their baby's two week checkup, the baby is a few ounces under birth weight.

If you have been told that weight gain is not acceptable, look hard at this list of questions:

◊ Is your baby peeing and pooping well?

◊ Are your baby's eyes bright and alert?

◊ Is your baby moving its arms and legs vigorously?

◊ Is your baby meeting developmental milestones?

◊ Yes, your baby sleeps a lot, but when your baby is awake does he have periods of being very alert?

How tall is mom?

If someone were to ask you what weight a 33-year-old man should be, you would laugh. The range of possibilities varies according to height, bone structure, ethnicity and many other factors. Yet babies are expected to fit onto charts distributed throughout the country with no regard to genetics, feeding choice or almost anything else.

If there are nursing problems, the first answer should never be supplementation but must be to find the best advice and help available. Find quality help in person if possible and online if needed. There is nothing better than having an experienced breastfeeding expert watch you and your baby and give you the help and encouragement and support you need and deserve.

Too many mothers and babies lose the breastfeeding experience and the lifesaving and illness preventing benefits because we doctors are trained to look harder at the scale than we are at the baby.

© www.drjaygordon.com. Adapted and reproduced with kind permission

BREASTFEEDING IN THE LONGER TERM

Duration of Breastfeeding

The World Health Organisation recommends breastfeeding exclusively for the first six months; that breastmilk be the main source of food for the first twelve months; and that breastfeeding continue for at least the first two years and thereafter as long as the mother and child desire. While that might seem like an awfully long time, bear in mind that, as a baby gets older, she will not nurse as frequently, or for as long, as a newborn baby. Most toddler nurslings will only breastfeed first thing in the morning, last thing at night and perhaps on one or two other occasions during the day. Play it by ear and see what suits you and your baby. Breastmilk is liquid love and the more of it you can give your baby the better.

For guidelines on your rights as a breastfeeding mother in employment, see Appendix B, pages 241–242.

The Milk Bank

If your supply is plentiful, you might consider donating your spare milk to the milk bank. The milk bank is a place where human milk is collected, processed and stored. This milk is made available to sick babies in hospitals and other specialist baby units throughout Ireland. By donating milk to the bank you are helping tiny, premature, sick babies survive and leave hospital more quickly. For further information, contact the milk bank directly at (048) 68628333 or e-mail milkbank@sperrinlakeland. freeserve.co.uk. There has also been a new worldwide movement of breastmilk "sharing" where mums with an oversupply provide their breastmilk to mums who are having problems breastfeeding.

Breastfeeding Support

If you find breastfeeding difficult, there are many people who can help and reassure you:

◊ At the Hospital or at Home. The midwife should have experience with breastfeeding mothers and will be able to help you get started. Some are lactation consultants and have specific training in breastfeeding support. In addition, most hospitals run a weekly drop-in breastfeeding clinic. Some Public Health Nurses also run weekly breastfeeding clinics but be warned that these can become baby "weightwatchers" and advice can be inconsistent.

◊ At the Local Health Centre. Breastfeeding support groups are run by the public health nurse. Meetings take place weekly, where you and other mothers can meet the nurse to discuss any problems you might have and to seek her advice.

◊ Breastfeeding Counsellors. Cuidiu, The Irish Childbirth Trust, has a list of trained breastfeeding counsellors who will answer any queries you might have. They are available all over the country. Contact Cuidiu for the name of your nearest counsellor. In addition, the La Leche League is a voluntary group which provides information and support to women who want to breastfeed their babies. Their services include telephone counselling, monthly group meetings and a referral service to GPs and Public Health Nurses. A list of La Leche League counsellors (or "leaders") is provided in the telephone book under "La Leche League". Telephone the counsellor nearest you.

◊ Breastfeeding Support Groups. Both Cuidiu and La Leche League organise breastfeeding support groups. Contact them for the number of your nearest group. Most breastfeeding support services are available free of charge although Cuidiu and the La Leche League charge a small annual membership fee.

© www.parentingweb.com. Adapted and reproduced with kind permission.

Kangaroo Care

A baby kangaroo isn't quite ready for the world when it is born but nature has devised the perfect way for the joey to thrive outside the womb with skin to skin contact with its mother. **Kangaroo care** is a way of holding a premature baby so that there is skin-to-skin contact, usually between the mother and baby — or father and baby when mum is resting. Your baby wears only a nappy, and is held upright against your bare chest. Kangaroo care has been shown to improve a premature baby's breathing and regulate his body temperature by skin-to-skin contact, and he gets the benefit of easy access to your breasts. If you give birth prematurely, check with your hospital to see if they encourage kangaroo care. Research is very supportive of this therapy.

Infant Massage

Mothers in other cultures massage their babies regularly. It is a won-derful way of connecting with your baby, helping him to ad-just to life outside the womb while also lowering your own stress levels. It's a lovely routine to get into after bathtime and can help your baby sleep better (don't we all sleep better after a nice mas-sage!).

According to wwwhomebirth.ie, the benefits of infant mas-sage include:

◊ Helps the parents and baby bond

◊ You become more confident handling your baby and reading his cues (non-verbal communication)

◊ It's a great way for dads to connect with their baby in the eve-nings if they've been gone all day.

For the baby the benefits are numerous; it helps with:

◊ Digestion

◊ The circulatory system

◊ It calms and relaxes your baby.

There are several books about baby massage but for some taking a class is helpful, and you'll get to meet other mums. During the class the instructor demonstrates the movements to the class on a doll, with each parent following along massaging their own baby.

Infant massage is fun and enjoyable for both parent and baby. You can massage your baby from a very early age; there is now evidence that shows that sick or premature babies benefit from "touch" massage (McClure, 1998).

Taking Care of Yourself After the Birth

In an ideal world, your partner would be a teacher (a well-paid one) and you would give birth a week after the school summer holidays started. Then you and your new family would have two picture-perfect sun-filled months together, bonding and cooing over each other. Well, for those of us who aren't so lucky, the realities of those first few days and weeks can be the stuff that nightmares are made of.

Coming home with your newborn (especially if this is your first) is an exciting but terrifying trip. First of all, you can't quite believe that they are letting you leave with this little baby; you are half-expecting an alarm to go off as you walk out the hospital doors. You find yourself driving like a learner again and all of a sudden everyone else on the road is an irresponsible driver.

The first thing to do when you get home? Get into your pjs and go to bed with your baby. Let everyone know that you're dying to show off your baby but you'd only like to have visitors in the evening/morning (whatever suits you). It's your partner's job for the next few days while you're off to make sure that you do nothing more than snuggle in bed and feed your baby. If your partner isn't Jamie Oliver, then make up a few casseroles in the run-up to your due date and freeze them so you have instant home-cooked meals at the ready.

YOUR BODY

You've escaped having periods for nine months; after birth, you'll make up for that with about six weeks of what's known as lochia (a bloody discharge) that will go on for a few weeks. It'll start off bright red and eventually turn brown, and then yellow. You won't want to look at tampons, so stick with the heavy duty pads with wings or maternity pads.

If you've had an episiotomy or have a tear (with or without stitches), whatever you do don't even think of getting a mirror out for at least a week. You won't recognise your privates, so best to remember them as they were! A few times a day, put a little warm water in the tub or into a basin and sit in it; it will help with healing and feels wonderful. Homeopathic arnica (taken orally) is reported (by mothers, not research) to be really helpful in reducing swelling.

Sometimes the extra pressure in the pelvic area combined with a long second stage of labour (pushing) can result in piles (haemorrhoids) – another good reason to leave the mirror in your makeup bag for at least a week. The good news is they will get better . . . eventually.

It will take a few weeks before you get into a routine with your baby. Don't expect everything to fall into place immediately. You're getting to know your baby and your baby is getting to know you. Take any and all offers of help! Sleep when your baby sleeps. Don't fall into the trap of trying to get caught up on cleaning the house or doing laundry. There will always be clothes to wash and plates to clean but these precious days with your new baby won't last forever. Enjoy them!

YOUR EMOTIONS

The kind of birth you have and your feelings about it will affect your transition to parenthood either positively or negatively. It can also affect breastfeeding. So often we hear, usually from well-meaning friends, that the birth experience doesn't really matter and are told "just be grateful you have a healthy baby". But that doesn't help if you didn't have the experience you were expecting. If you or a mother you know is having a hard time dealing with a birth experience, encourage them to talk about it or write down their birth story.

Sometimes being at home with a newborn all day can be isolating, especially if you don't have much family around and all your friends are at work. Check you local community centre for mother and baby gatherings or contact Cuidiu for mum and baby groups near you.

Postnatal Depression

Postnatal depression, like ordinary depression, is not always easy to detect, and is difficult to distinguish from the "baby blues", which will usually dissipate over time. Usually, some or all of the following symptoms will persist for at least two weeks in PND:

◊ Mood swings

◊ "Weepiness" and generally "low" feelings

◊ Feeling like you're not cut out to be a mother

◊ Poor self-esteem and self-image

◊ Lack of appetite or, conversely, comfort eating

◊ Recurrent thoughts about self-harm, death or suicide

◊ Detachment from reality

◊ Inability to connect emotionally with family, especially the new baby.

Discovery Home and Health (www.discoveryhealth.co.uk) states that the risk of becoming depressed within five weeks of delivery is three times greater than the risk of depression in the general population. It can happen to any woman who has had a baby, and certain things are known to make it more likely:

◊ A difficult, traumatic delivery

◊ Difficult home relationships

◊ Lack of social support

◊ Adverse life events

◊ A past history of depression or postnatal depression.

Preventing and Coping with PND

We don't know enough about PND to prevent it in the first place, but certain principles make sense.

Before the birth:

◊ Do make friends with other couples who are expecting or have just had a baby; among other things, it makes life easier knowing that other couples are trying to adjust to parenthood just like you are

◊ Don't try to be a superwoman. Having a baby may be a full-time occupation, so try to reduce commitments during your pregnancy. (If you are at work, make sure you get regular and sufficient nourishment and put your feet up during the lunch hour.)

◊ Do identify someone in whom you can confide. It helps so much to have a close friend you can turn to. (If you can't easily find someone, try the PND Association of Ireland, or Cuidiu, the Irish Childbirth Trust; their local groups are very supportive before and after childbirth.)

◊ Don't move house (if you can help it) while you are pregnant or until the baby is six months old.

◊ Do go to antenatal classes – and take your partner with you!

If you have suffered from PND before, that doesn't mean that you will do so again. However, it is only sensible to keep in touch with your GP (and, after the birth, your Health Visitor) so that, should there be any signs of recurrence, treatment can start at once.

After the baby has arrived:

◊ Do take every opportunity to get your head down. Try to learn the knack of cat-napping. Your partner can give the baby a bottle-feed at night, using your own expressed milk if you like. (If you're breastfeeding, try not to introduce a bottle for about six weeks to avoid nipple confusion.)

◊ Don't blame yourself or him: life is tough at this time, and tiredness and irritability on both sides can lead to quarrels. But "having a go" at each other may weaken your relationship when it needs to be at its strongest.

◊ Do get enough nourishment. Healthy foods like salads, fresh vegetables, fruit, fruit juices, milk and cereals are all nice, packed with vitamins and don't need much cooking.

◊ Don't be afraid to ask for help.

◊ Do find the time to have fun with your partner. Try to find a babysitter and get out together for a meal, a show, to see friends or just visit the pub.

◊ Do let yourself and your partner be intimate, even if you don't yet feel like sex: at least kiss and cuddle. This will comfort you both and lead all the sooner to the return of full sexual feeling.

Finally even if the PND is well established by the time it is recognised, support, counselling and medication will often make a big difference and will speed up eventual recovery: It's never too late!

How partners/family/friends can help

For family and friends:

◊ Encourage the depressed mother to seek help from a GP, public health nurse or counsellor.

◊ Encourage her to join a support group. Social isolation can contribute to postnatal depression.

◊ Try to be patient.

◊ Assist in arranging practical child care.

◊ Try to let her express her true feelings and treat them with sympathy.

◊ Try to find out more about postnatal depression.

Especially for fathers:

◊ Try, as a couple, to go out without the children, but don't force her to do anything she doesn't feel ready for.

◊ Frequently assure her that her illness is temporary and that she will get well.

◊ Encourage activity, even though she might resist, e.g. you might suggest going for a walk together.

◊ Try to ensure that your partner gets enough food and rest.

◊ Give her a massage – this will help her relax and restore her well-being.

◊ Reassure her of your support and that you will not abandon her.

Postnatal depression threatens the mother's and father's health, marriage, friendship and career, as well as the baby's welfare. Dealing with issues on a day to day basis can be a special challenge for family and friends. With your support and patience you can assist the depressed mother's recovery.

© *Reproduced with kind permission of the PND Association of Ireland and the Royal Association of Psychiatrists in the UK.*

What Your Parents Never Told You about Becoming Parents

Most expectant couples will spend countless hours in antenatal classes learning all about labour and birth; then there's the yoga class, the breastfeeding class and then newborn basics. By the time the big day arrives, most couples are just ready to get the show on the road, give up all these classes and get on with the real business of having their baby. But as more seasoned parents will tell you, it's only after birth that the real "labour" starts. You've probably seen that all-knowing smug smile creep across your mother-in-law's face when you tell her how tired you and your partner are from a day of shopping for the nursery. You probably only figured out what that look meant six months after your baby was born – or else just read-ing this chapter is giving you an Oprah "aha" moment – so that's what she was so smug about. . . .

WHY DO BABIES CRY?

For first-time parents, changing the nappies and giving your baby a bath come relatively easy once someone has shown you how. But with smaller families and siblings living further away from each other than ever, many of us never get to hold a newborn before we hold our own. As for calming a crying baby, sometimes it's not as easy as it looks. We've come to believe that it's our fate and even a parenting rite of passage that we have to endure spates of endless crying.

Babies cry for more reasons than I can include here. It's their way of communicating, and the most common reasons are that they are hungry, wet, tired, sick or they just need a cuddle.

In 1962, Dr T. Berry Brazelton asked 82 new mothers to record how much their normal healthy babies cried each day during the first three months of life. Dr Brazelton discovered that at two weeks of age, 25 per cent of the babies cried for more than two hours each day. By six weeks, 25 per cent cried for more than three hours a day. Reassuringly, he found that by three months almost all were back to crying for about one hour a day. (Source: Dr Harvey Karp, *The Happiest Baby on the Block*)

Sometimes your baby may be diagnosed with "**colic**". A colicky baby will easily fit the following "profile": he will cry for three hours a day (usually evening), three days a week, three weeks in a row. It usually starts around two weeks of age and peaks at six weeks and is often much worse in the evening. Babies are healthy and happy between crying bouts.

While many experts have tried to find a pattern to this problem, there are no consistent links between the colic and a baby's gender, prematurity or food. There are lots of theories about why some babies tend to be more colicky than others but none really hold true when investigated thoroughly. Most parents of colicky babies share similar experiences of their infants writhing and grunting, not being comforted by feeding or holding, or they have a piercing cry like their baby is in severe pain.

The piercing cry of a baby immediately puts the parents' nervous systems on red alert. Your baby's cry is unique to your baby and was designed to get your attention – fast. How often are you told that you'll eventually figure out what each "cry" means? But that's little comfort to a new mum and dad with a screaming infant on their hands after a long day at work. Or no doubt someone has told you not to pick up your baby each time he cries or you'll spoil him. You can't spoil a baby! Ignoring a baby and letting him "cry it out" would be like leaving your car alarm screeching until the battery eventually dies! Your baby may only need to be changed – or he may need medical attention.

An Easy Way to Calm Your Baby

Dr Harvey Karp is a paediatrician and a child development specialist in Santa Monica, California. He has spent many years trying to figure out the mystery of colic and why it affects some babies and not others. Through his research he has developed an easy technique to turn even the fussiest baby into what he calls "The Happiest Baby on the Block" (www.thehappiestbaby.com). His highly successful method is based on four simple but revolutionary concepts:

◊ The Fourth Trimester: How to re-create the womblike atmosphere your newborn misses – outside the womb.

◊ The Calming Reflex: An "off switch" all babies are born with, which quickly soothes crying.

◊ The 5 S's: Five easy methods to turn on your baby's calming reflex.

◊ The Cuddle Cure: How to combine the 5 S's to calm even the most colicky baby.

Dr Karp believes that babies, especially in their first few months of life, can experience "fourth trimester" issues. Babies can have a difficult time getting used to the huge amount of stimuli in life outside of mum's body. Their reaction is to cry and cry.

The "5 S's" are:

◊ Swaddling: Tight **swaddling** provides the continuous touching and support your baby experienced while still in your womb. Other cultures have been doing this for centuries and "wear" their babies close to them. Interestingly, these same cultures don't have colic.

◊ Side/stomach position: Place your baby, while holding her, either on her left side to assist in digestion, or on her stomach to provide reassuring support. Once your baby is happily asleep, you can safely put her in her crib, on her back.

◊ Shushing Sounds: These sounds imitate the continual whooshing sound made by the blood flowing through arteries near

◊ womb. Did you know the noise level that your baby is used to in the womb is equivalent to a loud vacuum cleaner? The good news is that you don't have to ruin your appliances by running the hoover all day; instead, get a "white noise CD" which can be played over and over again. How many new parents break into a cold sweat when the doorbell rings after spending the last hour trying to put the baby down for his nap? I know I was almost psychotic – and my dogs would bark at the breeze! Babies are used to noise, so trying to soundproof his room to the noises of daily life (which he's used to listening to anyway) will just stress you out even more.

◊ Swinging: Newborns are used to the swinging motions that were present when they were still in your womb. Every step you took, every movement, caused a swinging motion for your baby. After your baby is born, this calming motion, which was so comforting and familiar, is abruptly gone. Your baby misses the motion and has a difficult time getting used to it not being there. Using a sling is ideal.

◊ Sucking: "Sucking has its effects deep within the nervous system," notes Karp, "and triggers the calming reflex and releases natural chemicals within the brain." This "S" can be accomplished easiest with the breast but a bottle or soother or even a finger will work too.

Not every baby will need all five techniques. Calmer babies will need only a few; fussier babies will need all of them. Gauge your success in calming your little one according to your baby's intensity. Like any other skill, it takes practice – my husband and I practised swaddling on a stuffed toy, and had it down to a fine art by the time Jack arrived. Dr Karp's Cuddle Cure may help make those first few weeks of new parenthood enjoyable instead of spending it desperately waiting to see that light at the end of the tunnel that everyone keeps talking about while you wish away those first fantastic weeks with your newborn. For more information visit www.thehappiestbaby.com.

HELPING TODDLERS ADJUST TO A NEW BABY

So you've sailed through the birth and now you're home with the new addition to your family. You've just settled down on the couch for a feed and your toddler looks up at you and asks, "When are we bringing the baby back?"

"We were so excited about the new baby that we didn't include Alex, our two-year-old, as much as we should – big mistake," says Gwen. "Within days of arriving home from the hospital, Alex had gone from sleeping through the night to screaming for hours and shoving our new addition Sophie whenever I tried to breastfeed. After the first day home Alex kept asking us when the new baby was going 'back' to the hospital. It was a difficult transition for all of us. I wish we had spent more time with Alex before Sophie's birth, preparing him for the changes."

Tips to Prepare Your Toddler

A new baby into the family is often the first major "trauma" that a young child experiences, especially a first and previously only child. This is a whole new world for him. Suddenly he's not the centre of attention anymore; someone cuter has come along and your toddler can't get a look in! For many toddlers acting the maggot may be enough to command your attention but in some cases a resentful toddler can resort to pinching or "cuddling" the baby a little too tightly – around the neck!

Your toddler's view of the world is fairly limited; he hasn't got a lot of life experience to measure this situation by so naturally his nose is going to be a little out of joint. Up until this morning he was IT; and in the space of a few hours (in his mind), his whole life has turned upside down. He didn't ask for this new baby and doesn't understand why you can't just "take it back". Time and patience is needed to restore his sense of security, which is the reason many young kids revert in their behaviour (start wetting the bed, wanting to nurse again or looking for a bottle, thumbsucking).

◊ Talk to your toddler about the new baby coming. Make it something for him to look forward to. Let him listen to your tummy and talk to the baby.

◊ Talk about all the things he'll be able to do as a big brother and how he will be able to help you with the baby.

◊ Tell your toddler that the new baby is going to bring a special present for him when he gets here. (Daddy, don't forget to go and buy it beforehand!)

◊ Try not to disrupt his routine with lots of changes all at once. If your toddler is getting close to being moved to his "big" bed, do it well before your new baby arrives.

© *Dr Amy Feldman; reproduced with kind permission.*

PARENTING STYLES

These days there are as many books on parenting styles as there are birth books, and just like your pregnancy everyone has an opinion on how to do it "the right way" (i.e., their way). There are several "trendy" styles of early parenting and I don't want to recommend one over the other because parenting is such a unique and individual experience. You will probably read a number of parenting books; some of the recommendations will sit well with you and some won't, but I can guarantee that your baby hasn't read them and won't know if you're doing "it" right or not. Follow your instincts and do what works for you and your baby.

> "No, he's not sick. He's not hungry, he's not teething, he just wants to scream. I'm doing everything I can but I can't please him. If he was 35 this is when we would break up."
> – Miranda from *Sex and The City* on Motherhood

Life with a newborn is intense – becoming a mother is intense – but you can't understand it until you live it and no book can prepare you for the reality of the adjustment that comes along with this new addition. It's a wonderful, amazing change but it can also be a frightening lonely change too. Things will never get back to normal again – you have a new normal and if you can let go of the reigns and go with the flow for the next few months everything is much easier. As a new parent getting enough sleep can be a chal lenge, especially if your baby isn't one of those "good" babies who sleeps from 7.00 to 7.00 from one week old. You'll be asked if your baby is "good". I wonder what "good" really means? Good usually isn't about whether your baby has robbed any banks recently, but is directly related to how long your baby sleeps at night. And during the day – is he a good "napper"? Almost every sleep "expert" suggests the CIO (cry it out) technique – leave your baby to cry himself to sleep. New research shows that extreme distress blocks the full development of certain areas of the newborn's brain and when babies that are left to cry it out don't learn to go to sleep they've learned that nobody will come when they are distressed so they eventually give up. Babies don't have the brain capacity to self-soothe – it's part of the brain that develops closer to 18 months. Babies are small for such a short time and using the mantra "this too shall pass" can be a great sanity saver.

If, however, at any time you find yourself overwhelmed by the task of parenting don't be afraid to seek help. Among those who can help are Parentline and Gingerbread.

The Evolution of a Mother

Your Clothes

◊ 1st baby: You begin wearing maternity clothes as soon as your doctor confirms your pregnancy.

◊ 2nd baby: You wear your regular clothes for as long as possible.

◊ 3rd baby: Your maternity clothes are your regular clothes.

The Baby's Name

◊ 1st baby: You pore over baby-name books and practise pronouncing and writing combinations of all your favourites.

◊ 2nd baby: Someone has to name his or her kid after your great-aunt Mavis, right? It might as well be you.

◊ 3rd baby: You open a name book, close your eyes, and see where your finger points.

Preparing for the Birth

◊ 1st baby: You practise your breathing religiously.

◊ 2nd baby: You don't bother practising because you remember that last time breathing didn't do a thing.

◊ 3rd baby: You ask for an epidural in your eighth month.

Your Baby's Clothes

◊ 1st baby: You pre-wash your newborn's clothes, colour-coordinate them, and fold them neatly in the baby's little bureau.

◊ 2nd baby: You check to make sure that the clothes are clean and discard only the ones the darkest stains.

◊ 3rd baby: Boys can wear pink, can't they?

Worries

◊ 1st baby: At the first sign of distress – a whimper, a frown – you pick up the baby.

◊ 2nd baby: You pick the baby up when her wails threaten to wake your firstborn.

◊ 3rd baby: You teach your three-year-old how to rewind the mechanical swing.

Activities

◊ 1st baby: You take your infant to Baby Gymnastics, Baby Swing, and Baby Story Hour.

◊ 2nd baby: You take your infant to Baby Gymnastics.

◊ 3rd baby: You take your infant to the supermarket and the dry cleaner.

Going Out

◊ 1st baby: The first time you leave your baby with a babysitter, you call home five times.

◊ 2nd baby: Just before you walk out the door, you remember to leave a number where you can be reached.

◊ 3rd baby: You leave instructions for the babysitter to call only if she sees blood.

At Home

◊ 1st baby: You spend a good bit of every day just gazing at the baby.

◊ 2nd baby: You spend a bit of every day watching to be sure your older child isn't squeezing, poking, or hitting the baby.

◊ 3rd baby: You spend a little bit of every day hiding from the children.

AND FINALLY . . .

Pregnancy and birth are huge events in our lives and naturally bring with them questions and doubts. During those nine months all we seem to hear in our heads every day are those "What ifs?" – so let's look at them from a slightly different angle.

What If?

◊ What if I have an easy labour and my baby has a wonderful, gentle birth?

◊ What if everything happens just as I hoped it would?

◊ What if I breastfeed easily?

◊ What if having a baby is the most empowering experience of my life and I relish every moment of it?

Appendix A: Guide to Maternity Units in Ireland

Ireland currently has no national maternity guidelines, unlike the UK or US. Each hospital determines its own guidelines and policies which may or may not be based on best available research. Following are the results of a survey by the Irish Childbirth Trust to help families make informed decisions about their care during pregnancy. There are significant differences in caesarean rates, episiotomy rates and induction of labour rates around the country. Visit bump2babe.ie for additional details on your maternity unit.[1]

Spontaneous Onset of Labour

Hospital	All Mothers	First Time Mothers	Second and Subsequent Time Mothers
Cavan General	–	–	–
Midwifery-Led Unit cavan	100%	–	–
Cork Univ. Maternity	–	–	–
Letterkenny General	–	–	–
Coombe Women & Infants	55.8%	54.9%	56.4%
Mount Carmel	44.6%	56.1%	37.7%
National Maternity	64.2%	61.4%	66.7%
Rotunda	60.8%	61.1%	60.5%
Portiuncula	64.7%	64.1%	65.1%

---

[1] Please note that stats for Cork University Maternity Hospital are not available at this time. Visit bump2babe.ie for the most recent updates.

Hospital	All Mothers	First Time Mothers	Second and Subsequent Time Mothers
University Galway	55.5%	56.2%	55%
Kerry General	56.9%	–	–
St Luke's Kilkenny	–	–	–
Midland Regional Portlaoise	–	–	–
Mid West Regional Limerick	52%	52.5%	51.6%
Our Lady of Lourdes Drogheda	59.5%	59.4%	59.6%
Midwife-Led Unit Our Lady of Lourdes	100%	100%	100%
Mayo General	64.4%	58.2%	68.2%
Sligo General	66.2%	–	–
South Tipperary General	68.4%	70.7%	66.4%
Waterford Regional	–	–	–
Midland Regional Mullingar	–	–	–
Wexford General	–	–	–

Labour Induced

Hospital	All Mothers	First Time Mothers	Second and Subsequent Time Mothers
Cavan General	26.3%	–	–
Midwifery-Led Unit cavan	0%	–	–
Cork Univ. Maternity	–	–	–
Letterkenny General	25.5%	–	–

Hospital	All Mothers	First Time Mothers	Second and Subsequent Time Mothers
Coombe Women & Infants	30.4%	36.9%	25.7%
Mount Carmel	27.2%	25.2%	28.4%
National Maternity	25.2%	30.7%	20.2%
Rotunda	23.3%	27.8%	19.3%
Portiuncula	21.5%	27.1%	17.9%
University Galway	26.6%	31.4%	23.3%
Kerry General	20%	–	–
St Luke's Kilkenny	21.6%	30.8%	17.7%
Midland Regional Portlaoise	–	–	–
Mid West Regional Limerick	31.2%	36.6%	27.5%
Our Lady of Lourdes Drogheda	22.7%	31.1%	18.3%
Midwife-Led Unit Our Lady of Lourdes	0%	0%	0%
Mayo General	20.7%	32.1%	13.7%
Sligo General	22.6%	–	–
South Tipperary General	15.8%	18.7%	13.4%
Waterford Regional	26.6%	–	–
Midland Regional Mullingar	–	–	–
Wexford General	–	–	–

Spontaneous Vaginal Birth

Hospital	All Mothers	First Time Mothers	Second and Subsequent Time Mothers
Cavan General	56.4%	–	–
Midwifery-Led Unit cavan	100%	–	–
Cork Univ. Maternity	–	–	–
Letterkenny General	62.2%	–	–
Coombe Women & Infants	57.5%	40.9%	69.4%
Mount Carmel	48.9%	36.5%	56.2%
National Maternity	65.2%	52.5%	76.9%
Rotunda	51.9%	37.4%	64.9%
Portiuncula	53.1%	37.1%	63.4%
University Galway	54.1%	37.4%	65.8%
Kerry General	54.3%	–	–
St Luke's Kilkenny	49.5%	–	–
Midland Regional Portlaoise	56.9%	–	–
Mid West Regional Limerick	58.7%	47.7%	66.4%
Our Lady of Lourdes Drogheda	54.1%	39.9%	61.7%
Midwife-Led Unit Our Lady of Lourdes	99.3%	–	–
Mayo General	60.9%	54.4%	64.9%
Sligo General	68.7%	–	–
South Tipperary General	47.7%	35.4%	57.7%
Waterford Regional	58.1%	–	–

Hospital	All Mothers	First Time Mothers	Second and Subsequent Time Mothers
Midland Regional Mullingar	63.4%	–	–
Wexford General	–	–	–

Spontaneous Vaginal Birth

Hospital	All Mothers	First Time Mothers	Second and Subsequent Time Mothers
Cavan General	15.2%	–	–
Midwifery-Led Unit cavan	0%	–	–
Cork Univ. Maternity	–	–	–
Letterkenny General	13.1%	–	–
Coombe Women & Infants	17.6%	33.2%	6.5%
Mount Carmel	11.2%	23.1%	4.0%
National Maternity	15.0%	25.3%	5.4%
Rotunda	19.8%	33.1%	7.9%
Portiuncula	18.9%	33.1%	9.9%
University Galway	17.4%	32.2%	7.1%
Kerry General	15.7%	–	–
St Luke's Kilkenny	14.2%	–	–
Midland Regional Portlaoise	14.9%	–	–
Mid West Regional Limerick	14.6%	27.3%	5.6%
Our Lady of Lourdes Drogheda	16.1%	29.3%	9.0%

Hospital	All Mothers	First Time Mothers	Second and Subsequent Time Mothers
Midwife-Led Unit Our Lady of Lourdes	0.7%	–	–
Mayo General	14.4%	19.5%	11.3%
Sligo General	13.4%	–	–
South Tipperary General	18.1%	28.1%	9.9%
Waterford Regional	17.9%	–	–
Midland Regional Mullingar	13.0%	–	–
Wexford General	13.3%	–	–

Caesarean Birth

Hospital	All Mothers	First Time Mothers	Second and Subsequent Time Mothers
Cavan General	28.3%	–	–
Midwifery-Led Unit cavan	0%	–	–
Cork Univ. Maternity	–	–	–
Letterkenny General	24.6%	–	–
Coombe Women & Infants	25.1%	26.2%	24.3%
Mount Carmel	38.7%	36.1%	40.3%
National Maternity	19.9%	22.1%	17.8%
Rotunda	28.5%	29.7%	27.3%
Portiuncula	28.1%	30.2%	26.7%
University Galway	28.1%	30.0%	26.7%

Hospital	All Mothers	First Time Mothers	Second and Subsequent Time Mothers
Kerry General	30.1%	–	–
St Luke's Kilkenny	35.6%	43.2%	32.3%
Midland Regional Portlaoise	28.2%	–	–
Mid West Regional Limerick	25.9%	24.4%	26.9%
Our Lady of Lourdes Drogheda	29.8%	30.8%	29.3%
Midwife-Led Unit Our Lady of Lourdes	0.7%	–	–
Mayo General	25.8%	27.5%	24.7%
Sligo General	18.9%	–	–
South Tipperary General	33.9%	35.5%	32.5%
Waterford Regional	24.0%	–	–
Midland Regional Mullingar	23.6%	–	–
Wexford General	20.4%	–	–

Episiotomy

Hospital	All Mothers	First Time Mothers	Second and Subsequent Time Mothers
Cavan General	16.7%	–	–
Midwifery-Led Unit cavan	0%	–	–
Cork Univ. Maternity	–	–	–
Letterkenny General	–	–	–

Hospital	All Mothers	First Time Mothers	Second and Subsequent Time Mothers
Coombe Women & Infants	15.8%	31.6%	4.5%
Mount Carmel	13.4%	–	–
National Maternity	27.1%	43.5%	11.8%
Rotunda	17.3%	30.1%	5.8%
Portiuncula	13.2%	24.9%	5.7%
University Galway	–	–	–
Kerry General	21.1%	–	–
St Luke's Kilkenny	17..9%	–	–
Midland Regional Portlaoise	–	–	–
Mid West Regional Limerick	13.6%	25.8%	5.0%
Our Lady of Lourdes Drogheda	14.0%	22.6%	9.4%
Midwife-Led Unit Our Lady of Lourdes	2.7%	5.7%	1.8%
Mayo General	15.8%	26.8%	7.1%
Sligo General	17.7%	–	–
South Tipperary General	15.4%	25.8%	7.0%
Waterford Regional	11.8%	–	–
Midland Regional Mullingar	–	–	–
Wexford General	8.1%	–	–

Initiated Breastfeeding within First Hour of Birth

Hospital	All Mothers	First Time Mothers	Second and Subsequent Time Mothers
Cavan General	58.0%	–	–
Midwifery-Led Unit cavan	67.8%	–	–
Cork Univ. Maternity	–	–	–
Letterkenny General	–	–	–
Coombe Women & Infants	51.6%	56.9%	47.8%
Mount Carmel	69.0%	–	–
National Maternity	63.2%	68.4%	58.4%
Rotunda	–	–	–
Portiuncula	53.9%	61.4%	49.1%
University Galway	59.9%	69.2%	53.5%
Kerry General	–	–	–
St Luke's Kilkenny	56.1%	–	–
Midland Regional Portlaoise	–	–	–
Mid West Regional Limerick	57.3%	–	–
Our Lady of Lourdes Drogheda	55.5%	59.5%	53.3%
Midwife-Led Unit Our Lady of Lourdes	66.3%	–	–
Mayo General	51.0%	67.2%	41.0%
Sligo General	61.6%	–	–
South Tipperary General	45.3%	–	–
Waterford Regional	52.2%	–	–

Hospital	All Mothers	First Time Mothers	Second and Subsequent Time Mothers
Midland Regional Mullingar	95.0%	–	–
Wexford General	–	–	–

Exclusively Breastfeeding on Discharge from Hospital

Hospital	All Mothers	First Time Mothers	Second and Subsequent Time Mothers
Cavan General	–	–	–
Midwifery-Led Unit cavan	60.0%	–	–
Cork Univ. Maternity	–	–	–
Letterkenny General	–	–	–
Coombe Women & Infants	37.8%	39.8%	36.4%
Mount Carmel	–	–	–
National Maternity	49.9%	52.9%	47.2%
Rotunda	47.7%	53.5%	42.5%
Portiuncula	48.8%	52.8%	46.3%
University Galway	31.7%	–	–
Kerry General	–	–	–
St Luke's Kilkenny	42.0%	–	–
Midland Regional Portlaoise	–	–	–
Mid West Regional Limerick	44.8%	–	–
Our Lady of Lourdes Drogheda	40.6%	39.5%	41.2%

Hospital	All Mothers	First Time Mothers	Second and Subsequent Time Mothers
Midwife-Led Unit Our Lady of Lourdes	53.7%	–	–
Mayo General	39.3%	49.8%	32.9%
Sligo General	40.0%	–	–
South Tipperary General	42.6%	–	–
Waterford Regional	51.7%	–	–
Midland Regional Mullingar	33.0%	–	–
Wexford General	–	–	–

Statistics for Home Birth with Self-Employed Community Midwives for 2009

Hospital	All Mothers	First Time Mothers	Second and Subsequent Time Mothers
No. of mothers books for home birth	150	33	117
No. of mothers transferred to care of local maternity unit during pregnancy	24	–	–
% of mothers transferred to care of local maternity unit during labour	33.0%	–	–
% of mothers who gave birth at home	93.0%	14.0%	79.0%

Hospital	All Mothers	First Time Mothers	Second and Subsequent Time Mothers
Onset of Labour			
% spontaneous onset of labour	100.0%	100.0%	100.0%
% spontaneous vaginal birth	100.0%	100.0%	100.0%
% ventouse/vacuum birth	0.0%	0.0%	0.0%
% forceps birth	0.0%	0.0%	0.0%
% artificial rupture of membranes (ARM)	14.0%	21.4%	12.7%
"Normal Birth" (spontaneous onset of labour, no artificial rupture of membranes, no augmentation, no epidural, no episiotomy, spontaneous vaginal birth			
Normal birth as % of all women attending unit	86.0%	78.6%	87.3%
Normal birth as % of women who went into labour spontaneously	86.0%	78.6%	87.3%
Episitomy/Tears			
% intact perineum	74.2%	–	–
% first degree tears	4.3%	–	–
% second degree tears	18.3%	–	–
% third degree tears	1.1%	–	–
% fourth degree tears	42.6%	–	–
Waterford Regional	0.0%	–	–
% episiotomy – instrumental birth	0.0%	–	–
% total episiotomy	2.2%	–	–

Hospital	All Mothers	First Time Mothers	Second and Subsequent Time Mothers
Third Stage			
% physiological third stage of labour	78.5%	50.0%	83.5%
% actively managed third stage of labour	16.1%	50.0%	10.1%
Breastfeeding (% of all mothers booked for care)			
% initiated breast-feeding within one hour of birth	94.7%	87.9%	96.6%
% exclusively breast-feeding on discharge	82.7%	–	–

Appendix B:
Government Guidelines –
What Are Your Options?

CARE OPTIONS

Depending on whether you have private health insurance, you may choose to sign up as a public, semi-private or private patient. Unfortunately, you can't mix the type of care you receive. In other words, if you want a private room in one of the public hospitals, you have to be under the private care of a consultant obstetrician – but even then there are no guarantees. . . .

Public Care

Every mum-to-be who lives in Ireland normally is entitled to free maternity care, covering antenatal visits, labour and delivery and postnatal care including home births. When you ring the hospital to make your first appointment, you will be asked if you intend to visit as a public, semi-private or private patient.

If you are a public patient, you will attend the hospital's antenatal clinic (or their local clinic in your community). You may see the same doctor on each visit, or you may not – it's pot luck really. Alternatively, if you have a fairly straightforward pregnancy, you can choose the midwives' clinic. You are far less likely to end up with a caesarean or routine intervention at the midwife-led clinic than if you're in the regular maternity ward. Midwife-led care is well documented to be the care of choice for mothers with no complications.

When you come into the hospital to give birth, don't expect your consultant to greet you at the door. The truth is, you may not even see your consultant unless there is a problem. You will labour in one place, then quite often play musical gurneys and move to the delivery ward, then to the public postnatal ward, so pack a light lunch; you'll probably cover quite a bit of mileage. Don't bother with the hospital tour – you'll get to see plenty of it when you're in labour (all joking aside, I highly recommend taking a hospital tour ahead of time). Chances are you will not have met the midwives or doctors who attend your labour and delivery. After the birth of your baby, you will be moved to the public ward for your stay, generally of about three days. A small number of hospitals now offer early discharge schemes, allowing you to go home early from hospital with follow-up care. If you feel you would like to be discharged a few hours after the birth, ask at your first visit if the hospital supports this.

Semi-private and Private Care

If you are attending as a semi-private patient, you may see a consultant privately, or attend the semi-private clinic. This clinic is run by the consultant and his/her team. In some hospitals a team member or the doctor on duty at the time may deliver your baby. After delivery, you will stay on a semi-private ward, with approximately 3–5 other mothers.

If you are attending privately, you will be assigned your very own consultant who you will most likely get to see at each of your appointments; you can request a particular doctor. Your consultant may not necessarily be available to attend your birth. Private care also entitles you to a private room, although, again, this is dependent on availability and as the birth rate continues to grow and hospitals continue to close, I wouldn't get my hopes up. It is also possible to find your own consultant; but do yourself and your baby a favour and don't choose one based on your best friend's experiences or from pregnancy message boards. This is one of the biggest decisions you'll ever make, so take your time and ask questions.

Maternity and Infant Care Scheme

You may opt for services under the Maternity and Infant Care Scheme, which is a system of combined care, split between your

GP and a maternity unit/hospital. The MICS service is provided by your GP and a consultant. You don't have to have a medical card to avail of this. Virtually all GPs have agreements with the health boards to provide these services; they do not have to be part of the GPs and medical card system. The scheme also provides for two post-natal visits to your GP. You'll have to get the forms from your GP and send them to your local HSE Area. You may need to follow up on your application.

Your GP provides an initial examination and probably a pregnancy test if you want one, if possible before 12 weeks, and a further six examinations during the pregnancy, which are alternated with visits to the hospital where you're planning on giving birth. The schedule of visits may be changed by your general practitioner and/or hospital obstetrician depending on your individual situation.

Around five extra visits will also be scheduled with your GP if you suffer from high blood pressure or diabetes. Only pregnancy-related complaints are covered at no charge. If you're dying with the 'flu and go to see your GP, it's not covered!

After you have your baby, your GP will examine the baby at two weeks and both you and baby at six weeks.

If you are having a homebirth the HSE will pay your Midwife €2,400 toward the cost of your homebirth. You will book in to your local maternity unit and be provided with the necessary scans/blood tests free as a public patient.

You are entitled to free in-patient and out-patient public hospital services in respect of the pregnancy and the birth and is not liable for any of the hospital charges.

Infant Care Services

The GP who takes care of you also provides care for your newborn. This includes two free developmental exams during the first six weeks following the birth. Your baby's entitlement to free GP services after that depends on whether you have a medical card. In other words, visits to the GP for any conditions related to the baby's health during this six-week period or afterwards are not covered by the scheme unless the parents have a medical card.

239

The public health nurse visits you at home during the first six weeks, which is a great incentive for new mums to try and get dressed before 4.00 pm!

Pregnancy and Employment Guidelines

Time Off Work and Antenatal Classes

Section 8 of the Maternity Protection (Amendment) Act 2004 allows you to take paid time off work to attend one set of antenatal classes (but not the last three of the series of classes, as these would normally occur after maternity leave has started). This entitlement is for one set of classes across all pregnancies while in employment. So, if you use your full entitlement, say, for your first baby, you don't get time off next around. If for any reason you are unable to attend some classes due to reasons beyond your control (e.g. pregnancy complications) you can carry over your entitlement to paid time off work to attend any untaken classes to your subsequent pregnancies (except the last three in a set).

Here's an example: you are attending a set of eight classes and this is your first pregnancy in employment. You are only entitled to be paid while attending five of those classes (as the other three would occur while you are on maternity leave). If for example, you become ill and cannot attend all five classes this time, you may carry over your entitlement to your subsequent pregnancies.

Dads get to come too! Fathers get to take time off to attend the last two antenatal classes immediately prior to the birth.

We all know that not all employers will share your joy about your upcoming birth and impending motherhood! So to keep the peace you're required to notify your employer in writing at least two weeks before classes commence, outlining the dates and times of the classes. If you do work for a David Brent, he could ask you for evidence of the classes (dates, times, etc.). If that's the case, I'd make sure to give him a play-by-play explanation of what a bloody show is and how terrible episiotomy is – he'll probably avoid you like the plague after that!

Employment and Antenatal Visits

If you become pregnant while in employment you are entitled, under employment law, to take time off to attend antenatal appointments. Similarly, you are entitled to time off for medical visits after the birth.

Let your employer know in writing about your pregnancy and if possible give him plenty of notice that you'll need time off to attend antenatal appointments.

If this notice is not given for reasons outside your control, then you can retain your entitlement, provided you write to your employer with an explanation and with the notice. You will need to do this within one week of the appointment. For any visit after the first appointment your employer may ask to see your appointment card. (Feels like being back in school!)

You are entitled to medical visits after the birth of your baby for 14 weeks following the birth, including any period taken on maternity leave following the birth.

Breastfeeding and Employment

Under Section 9 of the Maternity Protection (Amendment) Act 2004, certain women in employment who are breastfeeding are entitled to take time off work each day in order to breastfeed. The provision applies to all women in employment who have given birth within the previous six months. Employers are not obliged to provide facilities in the workplace to facilitate breastfeeding if the provision of such facilities would give rise to considerable costs. At the choice of her employer, the woman may therefore opt to:

◊ Breastfeed in the workplace or express breast milk, where facilities are provided in the workplace by the employer

◊ Have their working hours reduced (without loss of pay) to facilitate breastfeeding where facilities are not made available.

Women who are in employment and are breastfeeding are entitled to take one hour (with pay) off work each day as a breastfeeding break. This time may be taken as:

◊ One 60 minute break

◊ Two 30 minute breaks

◊ Three 20 minute breaks.

You should note that breaks may be longer and more frequent if agreed between the woman and her employer. Part-time workers are also entitled to breastfeeding breaks, calculated on a pro-rata basis.

Women who wish to exercise their rights to breastfeed in employment must notify their employer (in writing) of their intention to breastfeed at work. You must confirm this information at least four weeks before the date you intend to return to employment from maternity leave.

Employers can require the employee to supply the child's birth certificate (or some other document confirming the child's date of birth).

MATERNITY LEAVE

Maternity leave is not a "baby holiday", as my husband once remarked; it is time to help you recuperate, adjust to motherhood and bond with your new baby. It's a time you will look back on with fondness (those mornings spent cooing over your little one) or with horror (those days when getting showered by the time your hubby got home so you could prove how great you were doing was the highlight of your day). Some women complain that maternity leave goes by too quickly and others can't wait to get back to work, if only to have conversations that don't revolve around the colour of bowel movements and nipple confusion.

If you become pregnant while in employment in Ireland, you are entitled to take maternity leave for 26 weeks. At present, at least two weeks have to be taken before the end of the week of your baby's expected birth and at least four weeks after. You can decide how you would like to take the remaining twelve weeks. Generally, employees take two weeks before the birth and the remaining after the baby arrives! (Unfortunately, it's not just a rumour that some midwives may tweak dates so the mother can work right up until her due date. So instead of our legislation being forced to become more family-friendly, we are allowing it to become less family-friendly.)

The entitlement to maternity leave from employment extends to all female employees in Ireland (including casual workers), regardless of how long you have been working for the organisation or the number of hours worked per week. However, you do have to fulfil certain conditions before you are eligible to be paid for maternity leave – see below.

You are also entitled to take up to a further 16 weeks' unpaid maternity leave. If you can afford it – take it!

You must give your employer at least four weeks' written notice of your intention to take maternity leave. Get a medical certificate confirming your pregnancy. If you intend to take the additional eight weeks' maternity leave you must provide your employer with at least four weeks' written notice. Put everything in writing so there's no confusion or questions later.

It's not a bad idea to keep in touch with your employer while you're on maternity leave and you need to give him at least four weeks' written notice of your return date.

Public Holidays and Annual Leave

You are entitled to leave for any public holidays that occur during your maternity leave (including additional maternity leave). The right of employees to leave for public holidays is set down in Section 21 of the Organisation of Working Time Act, 1997.

Maternity Leave and Annual Leave

Time spent on maternity leave (including additional maternity leave) is treated as though you've never left the office, so you can still accrue holidays.

Stillbirths and Miscarriages

If you have a stillbirth or miscarriage any time after the 24th week of pregnancy, you are still entitled to full maternity leave. This means a basic period of 18 weeks and also eight weeks additional maternity leave. If you have satisfied the PRSI requirements, maternity benefit is payable for the 18 weeks of the basic maternity leave.

Postponing Maternity Leave

You can postpone your maternity leave in strict circumstances – that is, if your baby is hospitalised (not because it's the final week of Big Brother!). This right to postpone leave applies whether you are on paid maternity leave or on additional unpaid maternity leave. The maximum amount of time the leave can be postponed for is six months. You must notify your employer as soon as possible if you wish to postpone your maternity leave. Note that your employer has the right to refuse your application to postpone your maternity leave. The catch is that you have to have already taken 14 weeks' maternity leave first, four of which must have been taken after the birth.

If you postpone your maternity leave and return to work, then you may take your leave in one bloc, not later than seven days after your baby has been sent home from hospital. Again your employer can ask you for proof of hospitalisation and discharge after treatment.

If you postpone your maternity leave and return to employment, you need to notify the Department of Social and Family Affairs of this. You must notify them in writing that your child has been hospitalised and you have returned to employment. A letter from your GP/hospital is required to confirm to the Department that the child has been discharged from hospital and your maternity benefit should resume. Make sure your Personal Public Service Number (PPS) Number is on every document.

Remember, you may only apply to postpone your maternity leave if the baby has been hospitalised.

Illness while on Postponed Maternity Leave

If you have postponed your maternity leave and become ill when you return to work (before resuming your postponed leave), you may be considered to have started your resumed leave on the first day of your absence because of illness. Alternatively, you can choose to have your leave treated as sick leave.

Returning to Work

Yes, that day comes around for most of us! You are entitled to return to work after maternity leave and it can be hard on many parents. Your job is protected and if there have been changes while you've been away your employer must provide you with a suitable alternative. This new position should be reasonably similar to the one you left before materntiy leave.

You are entitled to be treated as if you had been at work during your entire maternity leave. Your employment conditions cannot be worsened by the fact that you have taken maternity leave, and if pay or other conditions have improved while you have been on maternity leave, then you are entitled to these benefits when you return to work.

MATERNITY BENEFIT

Maternity benefit is a payment made to women in Ireland on maternity leave from work and who have paid a certain amount of PRSI. You need to apply for the payment six weeks before you intend to go on maternity leave (16 weeks if you are self-employed). The amount of money paid to you each week will depend on your earnings. If you are already on certain social welfare payments then you will receive half-rate maternity benefit.

Maternity benefit is paid directly to you on a weekly basis into your bank or building society account. Some employers will continue to pay an employee, in full, while you are on maternity leave and require you to remit any social welfare payment to them. You should check your contract of employment to see what applies to you. Maternity benefit is a tax-free payment. If for any reason your claims are refused you can always appeal the decision.

Leave Certification

All employees must have their leave certified by their employer. However, if you get a P45 within 14 weeks of your estimated due date and you've satisfied the PRSI contribution conditions, benefit will be payable from the day after the date on the P45.

Length of Time Maternity Benefit is Paid

Maternity benefit is paid for 26 weeks. At least two weeks and not more than 14 weeks' leave must be taken before the end of the week in which your baby is due. If your baby is born later than expected and you have less than four weeks' maternity leave left, you may be entitled to extend your maternity leave to ensure that you have a full four weeks off following the week of the birth. In these circumstances, maternity benefit will continue to be paid to you until the baby is four weeks old. You need to notify social welfare by sending them a letter from your GP stating the date on which your baby was born.

If your baby is born prematurely before your scheduled period of maternity leave has begun, get your doctor to send a letter to social welfare (Maternity Benefit Section).

If you are employed you must have:

◊ At least 39 weeks' PRSI paid in the 12-month period before the first day of your maternity leave; or

◊ At least 39 weeks' PRSI paid since first starting work and, in general, at least 39 weeks PRSI paid or credited in the second last complete tax year before the year in which your maternity leave commences; or

◊ At least 26 weeks' PRSI paid in the relevant tax year and at least 26 weeks PRSI paid in the tax year prior to the relevant tax year.

If you are self-employed you must have:

◊ 52 weeks' PRSI contributions paid at Class S in the relevant tax year before the year in which your claim is made; or

◊ 52 weeks' PRSI contributions paid at Class S in the tax year prior to the relevant tax year before the year in which your claim is made; or

◊ 52 weeks' PRSI contributions paid at Class S in the tax year later than the relevant tax year.

If you are now self-employed but you were in insurable employment before you became self-employed, the PRSI contributions (Class A, E and H) paid by you in that employment may help you qualify for maternity benefit if you do not satisfy the self-employment conditions as stated above.

If you are already on a payment, half-rate maternity benefit is payable if you are getting any one of the following payments:

◊ One-Parent Family Payment

◊ Widow's (Contributory) Pension

◊ Widow's (Non-Contributory) Pension

◊ Deserted Wife's Benefit

◊ Prisoner's Wife's Allowance

◊ Orphan's (Contributory) Allowance

◊ Orphan's (Non-Contributory) Pension

◊ Death Benefit by way of Widow's?widower's or Dependent Parents' Pension (under the Occupational Injuries Scheme).

For new claimants, payment of the half-rate Child Dependant Allowance will be discontinued where a recipient's spouse's weekly income is more than €300.

Insurance from Employment in Another Country

If you were previously employed in a country covered by EU Regulations, and you were paying social insurance, you may have your insurance record in that country added to your Irish PRSI contributions provided that you have paid at least one full-rate PRSI contribution since your return to Ireland.

Disqualification from Maternity Benefit

Maternity Benefit will be stopped if you engage in any other work other than domestic activities in your own home.

Rates: How Much Am I Entitled To?

If you are employed, your weekly rate of Maternity Benefit is calculated by dividing your gross income in the relevant tax year by the number of weeks you actually worked in that year — 80 per cent of this amount is payable weekly. The relevant tax year is the second last complete income tax year before the year in which your maternity leave starts.

If you are self-employed, your weekly rate of maternity benefit is calculated by dividing your gross income in the relevant tax year by 52 weeks — 80 per cent of this amount is payable weekly, subject to a minimum payment and a maximum payment.

CONTACTS

For all information relating to government entitlements, visit http://www.oasis.gov.ie/birth/ Also, see the booklet Employment Rights Explained, Comhairle, 2003, a useful free booklet providing lots of information on employment rights, including a section on Maternity and Adoptive Leave.

The Equality Authority has responsibility for overseeing the implementation of the maternity leave legislation in Ireland. Queries about your entitlement to maternity leave, postponing leave, etc. should be addressed to: The Equality Authority, Clonmel Street, Dublin 2; Tel: 01-4173333; Fax: 01-4173366; E-mail: info@equality.ie

If you wish to apply for maternity benefit, you should contact: The Department of Social and Family Affairs, Maternity Benefit Section, Government Buildings, Ballinalee Road, Longford; Tel: 043-45211 or 01-8748444.

Glossary

Active Management of Labour: Protocol for managing the birth process through intervention, designed by the National Maternity Hospital in Dublin

Amniotic Fluid: The clear fluid that your baby floats in during pregnancy

Amniotomy: See ARM

Apgar Score: A scoring system that evaluates the newborn's well-being

ARM (Artificial Rupture of Membranes): Membranes are released artificially with an amniohook (looks like a crochet hook) instead of spontaneously

Auscultation: To listen to your baby's heartbeat

Bedrest: Confinement to bed on medical advice

Birth Plan: A written document to help you to define your birth preferences with your caregiver

Birthing Ball: A large plastic ball that you can use during labour as a comfort measure (also known as an exercise ball or yoga ball)

Bishops Score: A system of points that may indicate the success of an induction

Braxton Hicks: Sporadic tightening/hardening of the uterus (also known as warm-up or practice labour)

Breaking the Waters: See ARM

Breech: A baby that is presenting feet or backside first

Caesarean Section: Method of delivering a baby surgically through the abdomen

Cardiotogography (CTG): A machine that monitors your baby's heart rate

Catheter: A thin tube that is inserted into the urethra to drain the bladder when you have an epidural

Cervix: The opening to the uterus

Colic: A term associated with fussy babies that tend to have crying bouts in the evening for several hours

Colostrum: An important nutrient- and antibody-rich liquid that is present in your breasts before your milk "comes in"

Contraction: Tightening of the uterine muscles

Cord Clamping: Restriction of the blood from the placenta to your baby by a device (clamp) after the third stage of labour

CPD (Cephalopelvic Disproportion): A rare condition where the baby cannot be born vaginally due to the position/size of your baby and or due to malformation of the mother's pelvis

Dilation: The process of the cervix opening from 0 cm to 10 cm

Directed/Coached Pushing: Being instructed how to push (not mother-led)

Domino Scheme: Community midwife-run scheme that encourages home birth and early release from hospital (short for "Domicillary In and Out")

Doppler: A device for listening to your baby's heartbeat

Doula: A trained labour companion clinically proven to reduce caesarean rates

Eclampsia: The occurrence of seizures not attributed to another cause during pregnancy, usually after the twentieth week

EDD: Estimated Due Date

Entonox: A combination of gas and air used for pain relief in labour

Epidural: A method of pain relief produced by an injection into the spine

Episiotomy: A surgical cut to the perineal area to enlarge the vaginal opening

Evidence Based Care: Practices that are based on the best available clinical research

Expectant Management of Labour: A philosophy of care that adopts a wait-and-see attitude instead of routinely intervening in the normal process of birth

External Cephalic Version (ECV): A technique to manually turn a breech baby to a vertex position

Fetoscope: A device used to monitor your baby's heart rate

Foetal Distress: Reduction of oxygen to the baby, often indicated by consistent irregular heart rate

Foetal Ejection Reflex: The biologically normal spontaneous birth reflex which expels the baby, most commonly seen in an undisturbed birth

Foetal Monitoring: A method of determining the well-being of the baby

Forceps: An obstetric instrument used in assisted deliveries

Forewater Leak: Leak of the amniotic fluid in front of the presenting part of the baby

Guthrie (Heel) Test: Screening test on newborns to detect PKU

Hindwater Leak: Amniotic fluid that releases from an area other than the presenting part (membranes can spontaneously repair themselves)

Hypertension: High blood pressure

HypnoBirthing: An antenatal programme focused on relaxation and visualisation for birth

Induction: The process of artificially starting labour

Kangaroo Care: A way of holding a premature baby so that there is skin-to-skin contact

Kegels: Exercises to tone and strengthen the pelvic floor muscles

Labour – First Stage: Loosely defined as the initial stages of labour when the cervix dilates to 10 cm

Labour – Second Stage: The birth of your baby

Labour – Third Stage: Delivery of the placenta

Lactation Consultant: A professional trained in breastfeeding support

Lithotomy: The "on your back" birth position

Lotus Birth: The process of leaving the cord attached to the placenta and baby for several days

Meconium: A bowel movement that happens in utero or in the early days following birth

Membrane Sweep: A method of induction

Midwife: Caregiver specialising in normal birth

MLU: Midwife Led Unit

Moxibustion: A holistic therapy using heat and herbs, used to turn a breech baby

Multip: A woman who has given birth before

Obstetrician: A caregiver specialising in abnormal and surgical birth

Oxytocin: A hormone generated by the brain that instructs the uterus to contract

Pelvic Floor: The set of muscles and ligaments that support the uterus

Pethidine: A narcotic drug used in labour for pain relief

Pinard: A tool for manually checking heartbeat intermittently (looks like a little trumpet)

Pitocin: A synthetic hormone used to induce or speed up labour

PKU: An inherited genetic disorder that, if untreated, can cause mental retardation

Placenta Abruption: A serious complication where the placenta comes away from the wall of the uterus prematurely

Placenta Previa: A complication where the placenta covers the cervix

Placenta: An organ that develops in the uterus which draws nourishment in for the baby and takes waste from the baby

PND: Post Natal Depression

Pre-eclampsia: A disorder that occurs only during pregnancy and the postpartum period and affects both the mother and the unborn baby. Swelling, sudden weight gain, headaches and changes in vision are important symptoms.

Primip: A woman who is giving birth for the first time

Prodromal Labour: Normal pre-labour contractions before your labour really gets established

Prolapse (cord): Complication, often caused by ARM, where the cord comes before the baby and is compressed, possibly resulting in foetal distress and caesarean.

Prostaglandin: Hormone that stimulates labour (can be used for induction)

Psycho Prophylactics: Breathing techniques

"Rooming In": Keeping your baby with you at the hospital

Rubella: German measles

"Show": One of the many indicators that your body is preparing for birth; usually accompanied by some blood-tinged mucous

"Skin-to-Skin" Caesarean: A new approach to caesareans to make the experience more gentle for the mother and baby

Sonicaid: A handheld electronic tool to check baby's heart rate

Speculum: A plastic or metal instrument used to separate the walls of the vagina during a gynaecological exam

Swaddle: A method of calming a baby by wrapping him in a light cloth

Syntometrine (aka Ergometrine, Syntocinon, Synthetic Hormone Oxytocin): Used to deliver the placenta in a managed third stage.

TENS (Transcutaneous Electrical Nerve Stimulation): Device used for pain management in labour

Toxemia: see Pre-eclampsia

Transition: The point in labour when the cervix is between 8 and 10 cm dilated, where mothers often experience a lack of confidence

Transverse lie: Your baby is lying horizontally

Ultrasound: The use of ultrasonic waves for diagnostic and monitoring purposes for your developing baby

Umbilical Cord: A cordlike structure that attaches the baby to the placenta carrying oxygen and nutrients to the baby and waste way from the baby to the placenta

Uterus: A hollow muscular organ located in the pelvic cavity of female mammals in which the fertilised egg implants and develops (also known as the womb)

Valsalva: A method of directed pushing by caregivers

VBAC: Vaginal Birth After Caesarean (i.e. for subsequent births)

Ventouse/Vacuum: An obstetric tool used for assisted deliveries

Vertex: Position of baby is head down

Water Birth: The birth of a baby in water

Resources

Ante-Natal Classes: throughout Ireland.

Autism Support

Irish Society for Autism: 16 O'Connell Street Lower, Dublin 1; Tel: 01-8744684; Fax: 01 8744224; E-mail: autism@isa.iol.ie.

Baby Massage

http://www.babymassageireland.com/ Cork mobile: 086-1502136; Dublin mobile: 087-7557536.

Bereavement Support

Bereaved Parents Association, St Francis Day Hospital, Grange Road, Dublin 5; Tel: 01-8318788.

Irish Sudden Infant Death Association, 4 North Brunswick Street, Dublin 7; Tel: 1850 391391; General Enquiries: 01-8732711.

The Miscarriage Association of Ireland, Carmichael Centre, North Brunswick Street, Dublin 7; Tel: 01-8735702. Fax: 8735737.

Birth Pool Hire

Padraicín Ní Mhurchú, 36 Springlawn Court, Blanchardstown, Dublin 15; Tel: 01-8206940.

Naomi Clarkin, Brackloon, Westport, Co Mayo; Tel: 098-50830; Mobile: 086-3495728; E-mail: nomeandkillian@eircom.net.

Ray Thompson, 3 Carraig Mhor, Lott Lane, Kilcoole, Co Wicklow; Tel: 01-2872729.

Máire Reagan, 18 Fairgrove Dr., Bishopstown, Cork; Tel: 021-4342649.

Leslie Boal, Pinnhill House, Gortlee, Letterkenny, Co. Donegal; Tel: 074-26103.

Sarah Barry, Greenmount, Rathmore, Naas, Co. Kildare; Tel: 045-862048.

Birth Trauma Support

Anne Gill: Tel: 01-8450698.

Benig Mauger: www.soul-connections.com

Breastfeeding

La Leche League: http://homepage.eircom.net/~lalecheleague/help.html

Breastfeeding Clinic: www.breastfeeding-clinic.com. Enquiries to eileenosullivan@breastfeeding-clinic.com

www.ilca.org/ — for referrals to lactation consultants in Ireland

www.kellymom.com

Cuidiu (see below)

Cuidiu, The Irish Childbirth Trust

Cuidiu, Carmichael House, Brunswick Street, Dublin 7; Tel: 01-8724501, www.cuidiu-ict.ie

Caesarean Support

ICAN: www.ican-online.org

ICAN Dublin chapter: Tracy Donegan, Tel: 087-0572500

Caesarean Support Group: 111 Wedgewood Maples, Sandyford, Dublin 16. Tel: 01-2954953

Sligo Caesarean Support Group: Gwen Scarbrough (Midwife); Tel: 087-6710985; www.informedbirthireland.com

Vaginal Birth after Caesarean: www.vbac.com

Domino/Home Birth Schemes

Contact the Community Midwives at the National Maternity Hospital, Tel: 01-6373100 or 01-6373177; or your local hospital.

Doulas

Association of Irish Doulas: www.DoulaAssociationofIreland.com

Doula Ireland: www.doulaireland.com; Tracy Donegan, Tel: 087-0572500.

Doula Information (UK): www.doula.org.uk

Doula Information (US): www.DONA.org

Down's Syndrome Support

Down's Syndrome Association of Ireland: Island View Quay Road, Rush, Co. Dublin. Tel: 01-8439036

General Pregnancy/Parenting Websites

www.rollercoaster.ie

www.eumom.ie

www.thebabyorchard.com

www.mothering.com

www.babycenter.com

www.magicmum.com

Home Birth

The Homebirth Association of Ireland, 36 Springlawn Court, Blanchardstown, Dublin 15; www.homebirth.ie; Tel: 01-8206940; E-mail: homebirth@eircom.net.

Holistic Practitioners

www.holisto.com

www.homeopathyireland.net

HypnoBirthing

HypnoBirthing: www.HypnoBirthIreland.com (Tracy Donegan)

www.hypnobirthing.co.uk – for a list of local practitioners

Informed Choices

www.infochoice.org

www.maternitymatters.org

www.motherfriendly.org/

www.aims.org.uk/

www.cochrane.org

Lotus Birth

www.birthlove.com

Midwife Led Units

Cavan: Tel: 087-9799385

Drogheda: Tel: 087-2584951

Multiple Births

Irish Multiple Births Association: Carmichael House, North Bruns-wick Street, Dublin 7. Tel: 01 8749056. Email: info@imba.ie

Postnatal Depression

PND Association of Ireland: www.PND.ie; E-mail: support@pnd.ie

Aware, 72 Lower Leeson Street, Dublin 2; Tel: 01-6617211; Telephone helpline: 01-6766166, daily, 10.00 am – 10.00 pm; Fax: (01) 6617217; E-mail: aware@iol.ie

Parentline, Carmichael House, North Brunswick Street, Dublin 7; Tel: 01-8787230; Helpline: 01-8733500; Email: parentline@eircom.net

Mental Health Ireland, Mensana House, 6 Adelaide Street, Dun Laogh-aire, Co Dublin; Tel: 01-2841166; E-mail: info@mental-healthireland.ie

Prenatal Parenting

www.birthpsychology.com

www.prenatalparenting.com

Registering a Birth

General Register Office, Joyce House, 8-11 Lombard Street, Dublin 2; Tel: 01-6354000

Single Parent Support

www.gingerbread.ie

www.solo.ie/

www.treoir.ie

Yoga

www.birthlight.com

www.yogapregnancy.net/

www.yogaireland.com

Recommended Reading

Henci Goer, *The Thinking Woman's Guide to Better Birth*, 1999, Penguin (USA)

Sheila Kitzinger, *The New Pregnancy and Childbirth: Choices and Challenges*, 1980, Michael Joseph, revised editions by Penguin Books

Sears and Sears, *The Pregnancy Book*, 1997, Little, Brown (USA)

Sheila Stubbs, *Birth the Easy* Way (e-book)

Ina May Gaskin, *Ina May's Guide to Childbirth*, 2003, Bantam (USA)

Dr Michel Odent, *The Cesarean*, 2004, Free Association Books, UK

Kim Wildner, *Mothers Intention: How Belief Shapes Birth*, 2003, Harbor and Hill (USA)

Benig Mauger, *Reclaiming the Spirituality of Birth*, 2000, Haling Arts (USA)

Thomas Verny M.D., *Tomorrow's Baby*, 2002, Simon & Schuster (USA)

Granju and Kennedy, *Attachment Parenting: Instinctive Care for Your Baby and Young Child*, 1999 (USA)

Sarah J Buckley, *Gentle Birth, Gentle Mothering*, 2005, One Moon Press (Australia)

Nancy Wainer Cohen, *Open Season*, 1991, Bergin and Garvey (USA)

Suzanne Arms, *Immaculate Deception II*, 2001, Celestial Arts (USA)

Index

active birth classes, 65–6
active management, 40
acupuncture, 60
adrenaline, 84
amniotic fluid, 18, 71
amniotomy, *see* artificial rupturing of membranes
antenatal classes, 13–17
antenatal massage, 59–60
antenatal visits, 12–13
Apgar scores, 78
arnica, 75
artificial rupturing of membranes (ARM), 103–04
aromatherapy, 60

"baby blues", *see* postnatal depression
Bach flower remedies, 63–4
bedrest, 124–5
"big baby syndrome", 126
birth balls, 89, 147
birth partner, 42, 70, 90, 100–01, 109, 150
   choosing, 52–4
birth pool, *see* water birth
birth positions, 99–100
birth preferences, 54–8
   sample, 58
   why write them, 56
"birth show", 71
Bishop Score, 77
Boogie for Birth classes, 66
Braxton-Hicks, 22, 25, 93
Brazelton, Dr T. Berry, 216

breastfeeding, 198–208
   after a caesarean, 151
   benefits of breastmilk, 198–201
   duration of, 205
   support for, 206
   tips for success, 201–2
breech position, 33, 128–45
   external cephalic version (ECV) and, 143–4
   hypnosis and, 145
   "moxibustion" and, 144
Burns, Ethel, 60

caesarean section, 21, 55, 148–71
   care after, 153–5
   description of procedure, 150–52
   elective, 155–8
      birth plan, 159
   indications for, 148–9
   risks of, 152–3
   "skin-to-skin", 156
   vaginal birth after, see VBAC
cascade of intervention, 122
Cephalopelvic Disproportion (CPD), 126–8, 148
   relative, 149
Cheek, Dr David. 21
Childbirth Choices Today, 181
circumcision, 197

Coalition for the Improvement of Maternity Services (CIMS), 42
Cochrane, Archie, 34
colic, 200, 216–7
colostrum, 201, 203
contractions, 40, 69
cord, see umbilical cord
Cuidiu (The Irish Childbirth Trust), 14, 107, 173, 206, 211

Dick-Read, Grantly, 7–8, 10
dilation, 40, 58, 69, 78, 102, 104, 178
Domino scheme, 172, 176
doppler, 111
Doubleday, Jock, 181
doulas, 42, 52, 53, 79, 175

Early Transfer Home Ss-cheme, 173
EDD (estimated due date), 17, 76
endorphins, 59, 70, 84, 95
entonox ("gas and air"), 83
epidurals, 55, 58, 81, 108–10, 117, 121
episiotomy, 33, 58, 112–15
    myths about, 114
evidence-based care, 30–5, 93, 107
exercises during pregnancy, 66–7
expectant management, 40–1

"failure to progress", 102–03, 149
fetoscope, 111
Fisk, Nick, 156
foetal distress, 149
foetal ejection reflex, 119
foetal monitoring, 103, 111–12
    continuous, 111
forceps, 21, 55, 117–18

GentleBirth, 65, 92–8

Having a Baby Naturally, 5
heel prick test, 196
herbal remedies, 62–3
home birth, 176–91
    benefits of, 179, 183
    safety of, 180–83
Home Birth Assocation, 176
homeopathy, 64
hormones in birth, 84–6
hospitals
    choosing, 42–6
    what to bring, 74–6
hypnosis, 94–5, 145

Ina May's Guide to Childbirth, 5, 54
inductions, 41, 76–9
    methods, 77–8
infant massage, 207–8
International Caesarean Awareness Network, 166

Jones, Carl, 181

kangaroo care, 207
Karp, Dr Harvey, 217
Kegel exercises, 113
ketosis, 106–07

La Leche League, 203
labour,
    eating during, 105–08
    pools, 91
    positions during, 88–90
    premature, 72–3
    signs of, 69–73
letter of referral, 11
Lieberman, Dr Michael, 20
lochia, 209
Lotus birth, 186–8

MacLennan, Dr Alastair, 164
maternity benefit, 245–8
maternity leave, 240–4

meconium, 72, 150, 203
Mendelson's Syndrome, 106
midwife led units (MLUs), 55, 173–4
midwives, 12, 38–40
morning sickness, 61
multiple births, 123–5

Naegele's Rule, 76
Newton, Patricia, 15

obstetricians, 38–40
Odent, Michael, 188
oxytocin, 21, 78, 84
pain management, 80–101
Panuthos, Claudia, 87
parenting styles, 220–1
pethidine, 73, 82
pitocin, 78, 82, 151, 175
placenta, 18
    delivering, 192–3 see also third stage of labour
placenta previa, 148–9
posterior position, 145–7
    tips for turning, 146–7
postnatal depression (PND)
    preventing, 212–14
pre-eclampsia, 12, 123
Pregnancy and Childbirth, 5
Pregnancy, Childbirth and the Newborn, 5
prostaglandins, 78
pushing,
    coached/directed, 118–19
    learning how, 120–22

Remer, Molly, 87

Sears and Sears, 56
Sellick's manoeuvre, 106
Shanley, Laura, 5–10
Simkin, Penny, 5, 15
stem cell collection, 192–5
swaddling, 217

syntocin, 78, 82, 149, 151, 192, 195

TENS (Transcutaneous Electrical Nerve Stimulation) machine, 83, 91
tests, newborn, 196–7
third stage of labour, 192–5
Transformations through Birth, 87

ultrasound scans, 12, 17–19
    safety of, 19
umbilical cord, 18
    care of, 193
    clamping, 115–17
    prolapse, 104, 149
    stem cell collection, 193–5
vaccinations, 196
vacuum, 21, 55, 118
vaginal birth after caesarean (VBAC), 163–71
ventouse, see vacuum
vitamin K, 197

Wagner, Marsden, 31
water birth, 91, 188–91
    baby's experience of, 191
    how to use a birth pool, 190
Weed, Susan, 63
Wise Woman Herbal for the Childbearing Year, 63
World Health Organisation, 180

yoga, 65, 146